Register Now for Online Access to Your Book!

Medical Imaging for the Health Care Provider

Theresa M. Campo, DNP, FNP-C, ENP-BC, FAANP, is the co-director of the Family Nurse Practitioner Track and associate clinical professor at Drexel University, Philadelphia. She is board certified as a family nurse practitioner and emergency nurse practitioner with licensure in New Jersey, Pennsylvania, and Washington State. Dr. Campo works part time as a nurse practitioner in the emergency department in southern New Jersey. She has over 29 years of experience in emergency medicine, including prehospital, emergency department/quick care, and trauma. She received her doctor of nursing practice from Case Western Reserve University and her master of science in nursing, family nurse practitioner, from Widener University, Chester, Pennsylvania. Dr. Campo is a founding board member of the American Academy of Emergency Nurse Practitioners, a national organization, and was the inaugural chair of the education committee. She has served as vice-chair of the American Nurses Credentialing Center (ANCC) content expert panel for Emergency Nurse Practitioner Certification and was awarded the first board-certified emergency nurse practitioner (ENP-BC) in the state of New Jersey by the ANCC. She is a national and international lecturer on emergency and urgent care topics. In addition to *Medical Imaging for the Health Care Provider*, Dr. Campo is the co-editor of *Essential Procedures for the Emergency, Urgent, and Primary Care Settings: A Clinical Companion, Second Edition*. Dr. Campo has authored several book chapters and peer-reviewed articles. She is on the editorial board for the *Advanced Emergency Nursing Journal* and ReelDx (a video case study media). Dr. Campo was awarded the American Association of Nurse Practitioners (AANP) State Award for Excellence in 2011 and was inducted into the fellows of the AANP in 2015.

Medical Imaging for the Health Care Provider

Practical Radiograph Interpretation

THERESA M. CAMPO, DNP, FNP-C, ENP-BC, FAANP

SPRINGER PUBLISHING COMPANY

NEW YORK

Springer Publishing Company, LLC
11 West 42nd Street
New York, NY 10036
www.springerpub.com

Acquisitions Editor: Margaret Zuccarini
Compositor: diacriTech

ISBN: 978-0-8261-3126-3
e-book ISBN: 978-0-8261-3127-0
Image Bank ISBN: 978-0-8261-3159-1

Supplemental materials are available from www.springerpub.com/campo-medical-imaging

16 17 18 19 20 / 5 4 3 2 1

The author and the publisher of this Work have made every effort to use sources believed to be reliable to provide information that is accurate and compatible with the standards generally accepted at the time of publication. Because medical science is continually advancing, our knowledge base continues to expand. Therefore, as new information becomes available, changes in procedures become necessary. We recommend that the reader always consult current research and specific institutional policies before performing any clinical procedure. The author and publisher shall not be liable for any special, consequential, or exemplary damages resulting, in whole or in part, from the readers' use of, or reliance on, the information contained in this book. The publisher has no responsibility for the persistence or accuracy of URLs for external or third-party Internet websites referred to in this publication and does not guarantee that any content on such websites is, or will remain, accurate or appropriate.

Library of Congress Cataloging-in-Publication Data

Names: Campo, Theresa M., author.
Title: Medical imaging for the health care provider : practical radiograph
  interpretation / Theresa M. Campo, DNP, FNP-C, ENP-BC, FAANP.
Description: New York, NY : Springer Publishing Company, LLC, [2017] |
  Includes bibliographical references and index.
Identifiers: LCCN 2016039555| ISBN 9780826131263 | ISBN 9780826131270 (ebook)
Subjects: LCSH: Diagnostic imaging. | Image analysis.
Classification: LCC RC78.7.D53 C35 2017 | DDC 616.07/54—dc23 LC record available at
https://lccn.loc.gov/2016039555

Special discounts on bulk quantities of our books are available to corporations, professional associations, pharmaceutical companies, health care organizations, and other qualifying groups. If you are interested in a custom book, including chapters from more than one of our titles, we can provide that service as well.
For details, please contact:
Special Sales Department, Springer Publishing Company, LLC
11 West 42nd Street, 15th Floor, New York, NY 10036-8002
Phone: 877-687-7476 or 212-431-4370; Fax: 212-941-7842
E-mail: sales@springerpub.com

Printed in the United States of America by McNaughton & Gunn.

I dedicate this book to my husband Jonathan. You never cease to amaze me with your support, encouragement, guidance, and, most of all, love. This book would not have come to fruition without you! You are the reason I wake up in the morning, you are the love of my life, and you are my best friend and soul mate. God certainly blessed me with you.

Contents

Unit II: Interpreting Chest and Abdominal Radiographs

Unit III: Interpretation of Extremity Radiographs

Reviewers

David Angelastro, MD, FACEP
Director, Emergency Medicine
Bayfront Emergency Physicians
Shore Memorial Hospital
Somers Point, New Jersey

David Begleiter, MD
Clinical Managing Member
Atlantic Medical Imaging
Galloway, New Jersey

Kyle Deuter, PA-C
Certified Physician Assistant
Bone and Joint Institute of South Georgia
Jesup, Georgia

Dian Dowling Evans, PhD, FNP-BC, ENP-BC, FAANP
Associate Professor and Director of the Family/Emergency Nurse
Practitioner Program
Emory University
Atlanta, Georgia
Emergency Nurse Practitioner
Emory University Hospital and Emory Midtown Emergency Departments
Atlanta, Georgia

Johnny S. Gomes, DO, AAEM
Emergency Medicine Specialist
Frye Regional Medical Center
Hickory, North Carolina
Functional and Integrative Medicine
Physician, Director
Optimal Healthcare and Wellness PLLC
Morganton, North Carolina

Anne Hedger, DNP, ACNP-BC, ANP-BC, CPNP-AC, ENP-BC
Emergency Nurse Practitioner
Providence Newberg Medical Center
Acute Care Pediatric Nurse Practitioner Program Coordinator
University of South Alabama
Mobile, Alabama

Boris Libster, DO
Allied Gastrointestinal Associates, P.A.
Haddon Heights and Voorhies, New Jersey

Todd Luyber, DO, FAAEM
Atlantic Emergency Associates, AtlantiCare Regional Medical Center
Atlantic City, New Jersey

David G. MacBride, DO, CPE, FACEP
Medical Director
AtlantiCare Regional Medical Center
Pomona, New Jersey

Yatish B. Merchant, MD, FACC, MBBS
AtlantiCare Physician Group
Galloway, New Jersey

Aubrey Rybyinski, BS, RDMS, RVT
Lead Technologist
Navix Diagnostix
Taunton, Massachusetts

William Schumacher, DO, FACEP
EMS Director
Bayfront Emergency Physicians
Shore Memorial Hospital
Somers Point, New Jersey

Allen Lewis Silvey Jr., DO
Pulmonary/Critical Care Medicine
MedCorps Asthma and Pulmonary Specialists
Turnersville, New Jersey

Foreword

When the medical professional is confronted with interpreting his or her own x-ray studies, the task can seem daunting. In her new book, *Medical Imaging for the Health Care Provider: Practical Radiograph Interpretation*, Dr. Theresa Campo reduces the seemingly overwhelming task into manageable, logical steps. She literally takes you through the ABCs of interpretation. The information is relevant, practical, and immediately applicable to the modern medical provider.

If that weren't enough, Dr. Campo also is able to provide insight into the sometimes confusing alphabet soup of imaging, giving real-world guidance in how and when to order an ultrasound, MRI, and CT. By expertly explaining the hows and whys of imaging, she provides you with a powerful tool for understanding what to order for your patient, rather than reverting to a laundry list that you can never remember or never seems to exactly be applicable to the situation you are in.

These insights, along with a thorough knowledge of relevant terms and vocabulary that is so necessary in communication among medical professionals, makes this book one you will want to have by your side every day you are working. I know you'll enjoy and appreciate *Medical Imaging for the Health Care Provider.*

David Begleiter, MD
Clinical Managing Member
Atlantic Medical Imaging
Galloway, New Jersey

Preface

Welcome to *Medical Imaging for the Health Care Provider: Practical Radiograph Interpretation.* I prepared this book after I discovered a lack of suitable resources I needed to teach classes to nurse practitioner and physician assistant students in medical imaging and interpretation. I simply wanted to share the excitement I have for this topic with my advanced practice, interdisciplinary colleagues and help them understand the dynamics of the five testing modalities and approaches to interpretation of radiographs. I truly believe this book can be useful to all health care providers, whether students or practicing providers, in a wide range of clinical settings.

The intention of this book is to provide a concise, easy-to-use reference that introduces the reader to differences in medical imaging testing modalities and teach the basics of plain radiograph interpretation. It is designed to assist providers in identifying and understanding the various medical imaging testing modalities of radiographs, CTs, nuclear imaging, MRIs, and ultrasound scans and images. The book presents written descriptions of the various modalities that are enhanced with figures, tables, and actual patient films. The text demonstrates concepts and discusses in clearly presented language the various attributes of the range of testing modalities and how to interpret them. This approach helps to deepen the practitioner's understanding of the differences in the modalities, along with a deeper appreciation for the parameters of these tests, and supports appropriate utilization of these diagnostic tools when diagnosing patients.

This book is divided into four units. The first unit introduces the reader to the history of medical imaging and gives an overview of radiology and each testing modality. Guidance is provided on how to choose the best diagnostic medical imaging test to assess the presenting condition. Units II through IV cover interpretation of plain radiographs of the chest, abdomen, extremities, and spine. Age-appropriate considerations are included throughout the book, as is the importance of the clinical decision-making process. **The reader may also access the images and drawings found in this text at springerpub.com/campo-medical-imaging.**

Interpretation of plain radiographs can be challenging and frustrating for any provider, whether a student or novice. The simplified approach to interpretation is performed step by step utilizing the ABCs of interpretation. Having fail-safe measures in place, learning to interpret what you are seeing on the radiograph, and understanding the rationale underlying your interpretation will assist you in confidently diagnosing the patient. Whether you are reading a radiology report or interpreting radiographs, this important resource will help build your confidence in your ability to read and interpret radiographs. It will help you feel more self-assured and less stressed. So let's get started and have fun!

Theresa M. Campo

Acknowledgments

One person cannot move mountains or accomplish goals by himself or herself. My family, friends, and colleagues have helped me to accomplish my goal of publishing this book. I would like to say thank you for your continued support!

Dad, I want to thank you for the unconditional support you give me. You mean the world to me and I am so blessed with the relationship we have grown into. You are not only my father but a person I look up to and admire.

Atlantic Medical Imaging—radiology group—thank you for all of your support and guidance in developing and completing this book. Dr. David Begleiter, especially—thank you for all of your guidance, expertise, support, encouragement, and most of all the patience you gave me during the journey in completing this book.

Margaret Zuccarini and Springer Publishing Company—thank you for allowing me the opportunity to share my love for medical imaging with my colleagues.

I would like to thank the following individuals for assisting with illustrations and images. You were more than instrumental in making this book complete.

David Begleiter, MD
Clinical Managing Member
Atlantic Medical Imaging
Galloway, New Jersey

Douglas W. Parrillo, MD
Chairman, Department of Radiological Sciences
Drexel University College of Medicine
Clinical Service Chief of Radiology
Hahnemann University Hospital, Tenethealth
Philadelphia, Pennsylvania

Kyle Deuter, PA-C
Certified Physician Assistant
Bone and Joint Institute of South Georgia
Jesup, Georgia

University of Virginia

 Department of Radiology &
Medical Imaging

I would like to thank Heather Cox and the students from Ocean City High School who provided the awesome drawings for this book.

Heather Cox
Art Teacher
Ocean City High School
Ocean City, New Jersey

John Brittin Jr.
Jack Crowell
Matt Colbert
Andrew Haines
Paul Kenney
David Rosario

Introduction to Medical Imaging Including Radiographs, CT, Nuclear Scans, MRIs, and Ultrasonography

1

Radiology Basics

HISTORY OF RADIOLOGY

Having an understanding of not only how radiology began but also how it has progressed through time with the development of various testing modalities in the field of medical imaging will assist the medical provider in his or her practice. Radiology has been around for more than a century. It began in November 1895 when Wilhelm Röentgen discovered the Röentgen ray while in his laboratory (Figure 1.1). Dr. Röentgen was a Dutch physicist and was awarded the Nobel Prize for physics in 1901. His discovery came during an experiment with ray tubes where it was noted that a fluorescing plate portrayed an image of a hand with a ring on it. In the literature, there are conflicting reports of whether the hand was actually Dr. Röentgen's or the hand of his wife (Figure 1.2).

The Röentgen ray is invisible and able to penetrate objects, causing it to fluoresce. This ray was originally named by Dr. Röentgen as the *X-Strahlung*, which translates to x-ray. The first clinical x-ray was documented in 1896. Bismuth for stomach x-rays was discovered and utilized to contrast structures not readily seen on a plain radiograph. The dangers of x-rays were first discovered and documented in 1901. However, they were not classified as carcinogenic until well after World War II.

Numerous discoveries and "firsts" occurred throughout the 20th century including the modern x-ray tube in 1913, radiographic film in 1918, the automatic processor for film in 1942, and many others. Table 1.1 demonstrates the use of contrast material for stomach x-rays and barium used in the gastrointestinal (GI) tract. Other "firsts" during the 20th century included the first retrograde pyelogram, which was performed in 1906; the first cerebral

FIGURE 1.1 Dr. Wilhelm Röentgen.

FIGURE 1.2 The first x-ray.

TABLE 1.1 Historical Discoveries and Firsts in Radiology

Year	Contrast	Year	Discoveries	Year	Firsts
1897	Bismuth for stomach x-rays	1895	Röentgen ray	1896	First clinical x-ray
1910	Barium for GI tract	1913	Modern x-ray tube (hot cathode tube) by William Coolidge	1901	Danger of x-rays
1911	Double contrast for upper GI	1913	Stationary grid by Gustav Bucky	1906	Retrograde pyelogram using silver nitrate
		1913	X-ray film of nitrocellulose	1919	Pneumoencephalogram
1923	Double contrast for barium enema	1918	Radiographic film	1927	Cerebral angiogram
		1921	Intensifying screens by Carl Patterson	1929	Excretory urogram
		1934	Artificial radionuclides by Frank and Irene Joliot-Curie	1932	Nephrotomography
		1942	Automatic processor for film	1937	Angiocardiogram

(continued)

TABLE 1.1 Historical Discoveries and Firsts in Radiology (*continued*)

Year	Contrast	Year	Discoveries	Year	Firsts
		1946	Film cassette changer by George Schoenander	1938	Mammogram
		1946	Nuclear medicine		
		1949	Xerography (dry photocopying also known as electrophotography)	1941	A-mode ultrasound skull
		1953	Image intensifier	1948	Coronary artery angiogram
		1957	Whole body nuclear scanner by Hal Anger	1953	Technique for vascular puncture
				1954	Echocardiography
				1962	B-mode ultrasound
				1964	SPECT scanning
				1972	CT scanner
				1974	Positron emission tomography scanner
				1978	Brain MR image
				1980	Commercial MR scanner
				1985	Digital radiography, picture archiving communications and storage system
				1990	Helical CT scanner (spiral)
				1998	Multislice CT scanner
				2000	Molecular imaging

GI, gastrointestinal; SPECT, single-photon emission computed tomography.

angiogram in 1927; the first mammogram in 1938; the first A-mode ultrasound in 1941; and the first B-mode ultrasound in 1962. Nuclear medicine was first discovered in 1946, and in 1957 Hal Anger developed a whole body nuclear scanner. In 1964 the first single-photon emission computed tomography (SPECT) scan was performed. In 1972, the first CT scanner was developed and utilized, with helical scanning capabilities discovered and utilized in 1990. The first commercial MRI scanner was discovered and used to image the brain in 1978. As you can see, medical imaging has come a long way in well over a century and continues to grow and flourish as time continues.

With the progression from the plain radiograph to the CT scan, MRI, ultrasound, and advancement of nuclear medicine techniques, diagnosing and caring for patients has become more adventitious. Radiographs have assisted providers in identifying changes in air fluid levels, identifying masses, and finding other abnormalities, leading to a more definitive diagnosis. Godfrey Hounsfield invented the principles of CT scanning; with its continued progression into the digital age, this technology has allowed for earlier and more specific findings leading to not only earlier diagnosis but earlier interventions positively affecting outcomes. Ultrasound use began in the 1950s and has rapidly gained acceptance for its real-time images. It has been expanded from not only screening and diagnosis but also assisting in procedures as well as treatments to improve patient outcomes.

Radiology has rapidly advanced since its beginning in 1895. Having an appreciation and understanding of the history of radiological science and its discoveries allows providers to gain an appreciation for diagnostic imaging modalities while ordering and interpreting them on a daily basis in practice. An understanding of the testing modalities will also assist providers in choosing, interpreting, and utilizing the findings of the most appropriate test in caring for patients. This, coupled with the American College of Radiology (ACR) Appropriateness Criteria, can assist providers in remaining updated on how best to choose the most cost-effective and appropriate imaging modalities to reduce harm and improve diagnostic specificity.

X-Rays and Image Production

In order to have an understanding of radiographs and the images that are produced, it is important to learn what an x-ray is. X-Strahlung rays, also known as x-rays, are a form of electromagnetic radiation which, in combination with light, strikes a photosensitive surface; this produces an image that traditionally was processed with chemicals. The radiant energy, which is similar to visible light or sunlight, is a short wave that is invisible and can penetrate many objects and structures. The shorter the wavelength, the greater its ability to penetrate objects.

Quanta or photons are pockets of energy and are described in terms of particles that travel at the speed of light. Electron volts are a measurement of the amount of energy carried by each photon, which is dependent on the wavelength of the radiation. When an atom loses its electron it is considered to be ionized. Any photon with 15 or more electron volts is capable of ionization; this is known as ionizing radiation.

X-rays are emitted from a cathode tube. When the rays are released from the tube they are closely approximated but expand as they travel. The rays then penetrate a structure, striking a cassette on the other side. The amount of radiation that reaches the cassette after penetrating the structure is depicted on a scale from black to white defining the image. The amount of radiation that is able to penetrate an object is dependent on the amount that is absorbed by the structure reducing the amount of energy transmitted through to the cassette (Figure 1.3).

Traditionally the cassette held film, which would be processed with chemicals and hung to dry. The images, once they were dry, would then be viewed on a lighted view box or with a hot lamp. If a reading was read prior to it being completely dry it was referred to as a wet reading. There are still areas in the world that continue to use conventional film cassettes. However, with the

Screens — | — Film

(A)   (B)

FIGURE 1.3 Release of rays from a cathode tube forming an image (A). Note that the amount of attenuation causes either black, white, or shades of gray on the image (B).
Drawing by Ocean City High School student; image courtesy of Theresa M. Campo.

age of digital technology, the traditional film and cassette has been replaced with digital cassettes, which are processed by an electric reader. This technology has allowed for storing of digital images and sharing of digital images through a picture archiving communications and storage system (PACS).

Conventional film cassettes consisted of plastic sheets that were coated with an emulsion of silver bromide and iodide that was sensitive to light and radiation. The thin emulsion had a protective coating that, when exposed to ionizing radiation, produced a chemical change. The blackness of the film was affected by the amount of radiation reaching it after penetration through an object. If the radiation readily passed through the structure, the area of the film would remain black. The more radiation a structure absorbed, the lighter the structure would appear on the film. The spectrum from black to white on a radiographic image is determined by the amount of radiation absorbed by the density of the particular structure.

Digital cassettes do not use film or chemicals but rather photosensitive electronic plates that have computer-linked detectors; these read measurements of radiation striking various locations, which then forms an image. These images are stored and archived and can be shared by numerous providers at various locations, unlike traditional films that were kept in one physical storage location. This has allowed for viewing not only in various locations within a facility or between facilities but also anywhere digital information can be transmitted. Teleradiology is utilized by some facilities to allow radiologists from opposite sides of the world to read and interpret radiological images and report their findings. This allows for 24-hour accessibility, facilitating expedient results during after-hours and holiday situations.

Radiologic Density

As discussed, during the production of images, the amount of radiation that passes through a structure is captured by the cassette—whether film or digital means—thereby producing an image. The scale of black to white is determined by the density of the object, or objects, within the structure. The absorption of the rays by the objects is known as attenuation. Attenuation occurs through a process where the x-rays are removed through absorption or scatter during penetration of the structure (Figure 1.4). If the object is of increased density, then it has the ability to absorb the ray as it attempts to pass through.

FIGURE 1.4 Attenuation of x-rays. Drawing by Ocean City High School student.

There are two types of densities that are considered when discussing attenuation and image production in radiology: physical and radiographic. Physical density is the actual thickness and composition of the object or structure that affects the attenuation of the ray as it passes through. Radiographic density is the degree of blackness that is demonstrated on the radiographic image and denotes the contrast or differences in density of the radiographic film. Radiographic density of a substance is typically related to its physical density. Physical density can be influenced by the components of the object or structure. For example, the higher the atomic number and metallic component of the object or structure, the more it will cause a white effect in that particular area on the image.

There are four basic densities: air, fat, soft tissue, and bone/metal (Figure 1.5). These four basic densities correspond to the spectrum of black to white on a radiologic image. Air has a very low density that causes minimal x-ray absorption and produces a black area on the image. Fat produces a dark gray area and soft tissue produces a light gray area on an image. Bone that has a metal component to it from calcium produces a white area on the image. As the density of the object increases, that particular area becomes lighter on the image. The radiologic contrast between soft tissue inclusive of organs, muscles, ligaments, and so forth, is minimal to nonexistent since they are mainly composed of water. The greater the contrast between objects within a structure, the better the visualization of those objects. An example is air within a more dense cavity as seen on a chest x-ray of the lungs within the rib cage.

FIGURE 1.5 Four densities on x-ray. Courtesy of Dr. David Begleiter; diagramming, Theresa M. Campo.

The amount of attenuation corresponds to a unit known as the Hounsfield unit. Air that has little to no absorption has a designation of −1,000 Hounsfield units and is depicted as black on the image. Fat, which has minimal attenuation, is designated as −520 to −100 Hounsfield units and gives a dark gray appearance on the image. Water, which has some attenuation, appears gray on an image and is designated as zero Hounsfield units. Soft tissue appears as light gray on an image, since it has more attenuation, and is in the range of 15 to 60 Hounsfield units. Bone, which has a higher attenuation, has a Hounsfield unit at or near 1,000, and appears white on an image (Figure 1.6). Contrast materials such as barium or iodine-based products have a higher Hounsfield unit designation than water; however, it may be comparable or higher than bone. Therefore, they appear to be extremely light or white on the image. Contrast materials are discussed in detail in a later chapter.

1000
Metallic
Bone

500

Tissue
(15–60)

0

Fat
(–520 to –100)

–500

Air
–1000

FIGURE 1.6 Hounsfield units. Drawing by Ocean City High School student.

Since the discovery of radiology more than a century ago, numerous advancements and innovations have afforded better diagnosis and treatment of disorders. Understanding the science of radiography translates to better interpretation of findings. Knowing the basics of radiology and its shades of gray will help providers distinguish normal from abnormal findings and appreciate what they are actually visualizing.

FACTORS AFFECTING IMAGES

As discussed earlier in this chapter, it is important to understand what produces the spectrum of black to white and the shades of gray in between on a radiologic image. It is also important to appreciate what image effects are intentional or nonintentional. Adequacy of a film is imperative for an accurate reading of any radiological study. Nonintentional factors that can affect a radiological image can occur from physical as well as geometric factors, resulting in thickness, motion, scatter, magnification, and distortion. Intentional factors include those that are planned to highlight an area for evaluation with contrast enhancement.

Nonintentional Factors

The thickness of an object and its physical density can affect the attenuation of the rays attempting to penetrate that object or structure. The thicker the object, the more radiation is needed to penetrate that particular object. Conversely, the smaller or thinner an object, the less radiation is needed to penetrate that particular object (Figure 1.7). It is imperative that the appropriate dose of radiation be used to penetrate the object based on its thickness. If the same amount of radiation is utilized with a study on an 80-pound patient as opposed to a 500-pound patient, the image may be over- or underpenetrated. When an image is under- or overpenetrated, there will be inadequate contrast, resulting in a suboptimal image as key structures may fail to be differentiated and visualized.

(A)   (B)

FIGURE 1.7 Small (A) versus large (B) person.
Drawing by Ocean City High School student.

Another factor resulting in distortion is motion. Motion can result in a blurry or hazy image that may not be able to be interpreted. As an object moves, the penetrating rays become absorbed by the structure at different rates, making the image appear hazy or blurred (Figure 1.8). Motion artifact can be corrected with shortened exposure times.

Scatter is a deflection of the primary radiation beam and produces a foggy image (Figure 1.9). There are processes that can be used to reduce scatter and eliminate shadows that may occur. The Bucky–Potter system is a method that uses a grid with alternating angled slats that are very thin and radiolucent combined with thin lead strips. Rapid movement of the whole grid during exposure helps eliminate shadows and scatter.

FIGURE 1.8 Effect of motion causing a blurry image.
Courtesy of Dr. Keith Lafferty.

Magnification may be altered if an object is not the appropriate distance from the cassette. The farther away an object is from the film or detector plate, the greater the magnification of that object. This can reduce the sharpness of contrast, making it difficult to interpret the images (Figure 1.10). Magnification can also be altered by the direction where the

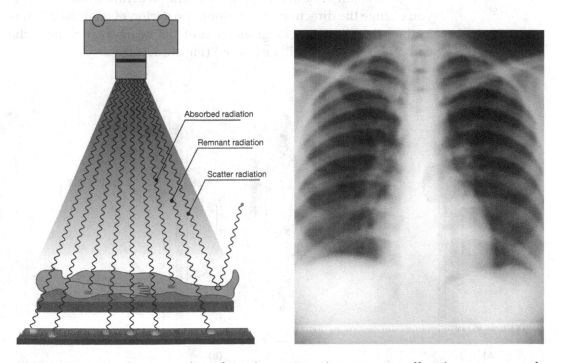

FIGURE 1.9 Scatter of x-rays causing a foggy image. Note that scatter can effect the appearance of the image.
Drawing by Ocean City High School student; image courtesy of Dr. Keith Lafferty.

FIGURE 1.10 Magnification effect on image. Note that the farther away an object is from the cassette the larger it becomes. The same is true as the beam travels through the body.
Drawing by Ocean City High School student.

ray enters and exits the structure. For example, in a posterior to anterior view, the beam of radiation penetrates the structure from back to front. If you change the direction to anterior to posterior, even if the beam is going in the same direction, magnification of the beam as it reaches the other end of the structure will be altered (Figure 1.11).

FIGURE 1.11 Posterior–anterior (A) versus anterior–posterior view (B).
Drawing by Ocean City High School student.

It is also important that the beam is perpendicular to the film or detector plate. When a beam is not perpendicular, distortion of the image occurs, affecting the clarity and appearance of structures.

Intentional Effects

Intentional effects of an image can be obtained with the use of contrast material. Contrast material allows for increased contrast of a particular object within a structure for easier visualization (Figure 1.12). Contrast may be used to examine structures that typically would not be seen on a normal radiograph. Contrast was used more extensively in the past in conjunction with standard x-rays before the invention of CT and MRI to evaluate abdominal, pelvic, or intracranial abnormalities. Contrast consists of elements such as barium- and iodine-based products that allow for better visualization of structures in radiographs and CT imaging or paramagnetic agents used in MRI studies.

FIGURE 1.12 Contrasted study. Note the ability to visualize the small airways otherwise not seen with a plain radiograph. Radiopaediageneral@radiopaedia.org

There are two types of contrast used for radiographs: barium and iodinated benzene ring solutions, such as gastrografin. Barium is used to visualize areas of the GI tract, specifically to better visualize the mucosa in detail. It is also beneficial in visualizing the luminal wall of the bowel. It can be given by mouth for an antegrade study or rectally for a retrograde study. Barium sulfate has a high atomic weight, which increases its radiological density; this causes a white effect on the film. It is resistant to dilution, which is why it is not recommended for the evaluation of large bowel obstruction or perforation. If the contrast remains in the bowel for a prolonged period of time, it becomes thickened and can cause the obstruction to become worse. It is contraindicated in perforation because it reacts with and incites granulomatous changes in the peritoneum. It can also interfere with subsequent studies such as CT scans, making them nondiagnostic. If a perforation is present, then the contrast can leak out of the bowel, potentially causing a desmoplastic reaction.

Water-soluble contrast containing iodide should be used if perforation or large bowel obstruction is suspected. Water-soluble contrast does not cause a desmoplastic reaction if leaked into surrounding areas and is absorbed and excreted by the kidney. The basic structure of water-soluble contrast is an iodinated benzene ring that also has a high atomic number, causing increased contrast and differentiation of structures not readily visualized on the plain radiograph.

Water-soluble contrast can be injected to highlight organs, vessels, and abnormalities. Angiography, myelography, arthropathy, and urography studies also use water-soluble contrast for indirect contrast imaging. Water-soluble contrast is contraindicated if an esophagoairway fistula is suspected or if one is at risk of aspiration, since leakage into lung tissue can cause a severe and devastating chemical pneumonia. If extravasation of the material occurs during intravenous infusion, tissue necrosis can result. Treatment for this adverse effect includes removing the IV catheter immediately, elevating the site, and applying warm or cold compresses to reduce swelling. If a large volume of contrast extravasates into the tissue, surgical intervention may be required.

There are many uses of contrast to enhance a radiographic image. Urographic studies to visualize the genitourinary (GU) tract involve administering water-soluble contrast either intravenously or through the urethra and into the bladder and renal pelvis, utilizing a retrograde method. The use of IV urography is replacing the use of CT scanning.

Angiography is used to image circulatory flow within an organ or structure. For these studies, water-soluble media is injected either intravenously or intra-arterially and then a series of images is performed demonstrating circulatory flow within the structure. A sonogram or fistulogram is performed to identify abnormal sinus tracts in the body by injecting contrast material within the suspected area. Inserting a needle between the spinal processes of the lumbar vertebrae entering the subarachnoid space and injecting a water-soluble contrast material under fluoroscopic monitoring is a myelogram.

One of the risks with water-soluble contrast agents is allergic reaction. Any persons allergic to iodine-based products should either be premedicated prior to the start of the study or an alternative radiologic evaluation should be considered to avoid a negative outcome. Allergy to shellfish is considered to be a risk for reaction to water-soluble contrast agents.

However, limited evidence shows an actual correlation. Patients with poor renal function or severe dehydration are at increased risk for contrast-induced nephropathy. Therefore, these patients should not be exposed to water-soluble contrast material. Patients who are dehydrated, diabetics, and those having borderline renal function should receive intravenous hydration before and after receiving water-soluble contrast, if an alternative modality is not available. Additionally, patients taking metformin with known borderline kidney functions are also at increased risk for a life-threatening lactic acidosis when receiving water-soluble contrast since metformin is normally cleared by renal tubular secretion.

Paramagnetic agents are used as contrast material with MRI, which helps to better define abnormalities and differentiate disease processes (i.e., herniated nuclear pulposis [HNP] from scars). There are two types of paramagnetic agents—gadolinium (Gd) and gadolinium-diethylenetriaminepentaacetic acid (Gd-DTPA). Free gadolinium is not used. Gadolinium gives greater detail to soft tissue and vascular structures. However, Gd-DTPA is the most commonly used paramagnetic agent due to its strong effect on the relaxation time during the scanning sequence. Relaxation time will be discussed in Chapter 3. Gadolinium has the ability to be mixed with iodinated contrasting agents useful in needle localization.

Adverse and allergic reactions rarely occur with paramagnetic contrast agents, and the risk of anaphylaxis and allergic reaction with the use of these agents is considered to be lower than those caused by iodinated contrasting agents. Nephrogenic systemic fibrosis is a rarely occurring adverse reaction that can occur with paramagnetic contrast agents. Nephrogenic systemic fibrosis causes a progressive tissue change in skin, joints, eyes, and internal organs that occurs more frequently in patients with renal insufficiency and failure.

CONCLUSION

Contrast agents can be very beneficial in differentiating structures with similar density that normally would not be visualized on an imaging study. They are also useful in identifying abnormalities such as masses, tumors, fistulas, and HNP, resulting in a more timely therapeutic intervention. Further discussion of the use of contrast agents with various studies is discussed during the chapters on the five testing modalities of plain radiographs, CT, MRI, and nuclear imaging.

RESOURCES

American College of Radiology. (n.d.). Appropriateness criteria. Retrieved from http://www.acr.org/quality-safety/appropriateness-criteria

Au-Yong, I., Au-Yong, A., & Broderick, N. (2010). *On-call x-rays made easy*. Philadelphia, PA: Churchill Livingstone, Elsevier.

Brant, W. E. (2012). Diagnostic imaging methods. In W. E. Brant & C. A. Helms (Eds.), *Fundamentals of diagnostic radiology* (4th ed., pp. 2–27). Philadelphia, PA: Wolters Kluwer/Lippincott Williams & Wilkins.

Daffner, R. H. (2014). Overview and principles of diagnostic imaging. In R. H. Daffner & M. S. Hartman (Eds.), *Clinical radiology: The essentials* (4th ed., pp. 1–42). Philadelphia, PA: Wolters Kluwer/Lippincott Williams & Wilkins.

Daffner, R. H., & Hartman, R. H. (2014). Radiographic contrast agents. In R. H. Daffner & M. S. Hartman (Eds.), *Clinical radiology: The essentials* (4th ed., pp. 43–48). Philadelphia, PA: Wolters Kluwer/Lippincott Williams & Wilkins.

Herring, W. (2016). *Learning radiology: Recognizing the basics* (3rd ed., pp. 1–7). Philadelphia, PA: Elsevier.

Taylor, C. R. (2015). Abdominal computed tomography scanning. Retrieved from http://emedicine.medscape.com/article/2114236-overview

2

Radiating Testing Modalities

This chapter introduces and briefly discusses the different radiological testing modalities that use ionizing radiation. The section on each testing modality describes how the images are obtained by the various machines and technology, their uses and benefits, as well as downfalls associated with each modality. This allows for differentiating the various modalities, but also gives an appreciation for how the images are produced. Knowledge of the various testing modalities is fundamental in understanding the most cost-effective and appropriate diagnostic studies for suspected conditions.

RADIOGRAPHS

Radiographs have been used for more than a century, revolutionizing current medical imaging. Since their invention in 1895, radiographs have been used to identify and diagnose abnormalities so that treatments can be given. The increased use of radiographs has improved lives through early detection of conditions leading to further studies and/or treatments of identified diseases. Radiology science has led to the development of more precise testing modalities such as CT, MRI, nuclear medicine, and ultrasonography.

Radiographs can be either plain, meaning there is no contrast enhancement, or they can be a contrasted study (Figure 2.1). Plain radiographs are ideal for identifying gross abnormalities and foreign bodies, visualizing calculi and fractures, or evaluating air fluid and gas patterns. They are advantageous because they are inexpensive, nonoperator dependent, and readily available as they can be obtained in a designated radiology room, using a portable machine, or in a mobile unit such as a mobile mammography bus. One of the disadvantages of radiography is its limited ability to contrast densities of organs and tissue.

(A)   (B)

FIGURE 2.1 Plain versus contrasted study. Plain radiograph (A); contrast radiograph (B). Notice how the contrast highlights the airways that are normally not visualized on plain film.
Courtesy of Associate Professor Frank Gaillard, Radiopaedia.org.

Radiographs are performed utilizing a single view. This means that the x-rays are emitted from the cathode tube and directed toward a cassette on the other side of the patient. The direction of the beam penetrating the patient is how that particular view is labeled. When we have a posterior–anterior (PA) view, the tube is behind the patient (or posterior, hence "P") who is standing or sitting erect with the cassette directly in front of him or her. The x-ray beam then travels from the tube, penetrating from the back to the front (or anterior, hence "A") of the patient. The image is then produced on the cassette in front of the patient (Figure 2.2A). In the anterior–posterior (AP) view, the opposite occurs (Figure 2.2B). The image is also labeled based on the position of the patient, such as erect, supine, prone, or decubitus. In the lateral decubitus view, the patient lies on his or her side for at least 3 to 5 minutes to allow any free air to rise and is then imaged in a side-lying position (Figure 2.2C).

FIGURE 2.2 Normal chest posterior–anterior view (A); normal chest lateral view (B); and decubitus view (C). Note the air/fluid levels on the decubitus view.

(A) and (B) courtesy of Theresa M. Campo; (c) courtesy of Dr. Keith Lafferty.

Contrast can be used to highlight areas of interest such as the intestines, bladder, kidneys, vessels, and so on. Contrasted studies can be static or dynamic. Static images are stationary images in a one-plain view. Dynamic images give real-time radiographic visualization of moving anatomical structures such as the heart and diaphragm. These are performed using fluoroscopy, which can be either diagnostic or therapeutic. Therapeutic uses can include cardiac catheterization with stent placements, injections into the spinal canal, or vascular line placements.

Fluoroscopy involves a fluoroscopic screen combined with an electronic device that converts visible light into an electron score stream. This technique amplifies the image, making it brighter, and then converts it back into visible light. When fluoroscopy is performed, the x-ray tube lies beneath the table. With the tube beneath the table, the cassette is then supported over the top of the table and the patient is positioned for the particular study or therapeutic intervention (Figure 2.3). The study may be labeled on the basis of the patient's position relative to the tube. For example, a right posterior oblique indicates the patient lying with his or her right side down, back against the table, at an angle greater than 0° and less than 90° with the tube beneath and the cassette overhead.

FIGURE 2.3 Fluoroscopic procedure table.
Source: https://commons.wikimedia.org/wiki/File:Fluoroscope.jpg.

Radiographs have revolutionized medicine since their discovery in 1895, leading to new testing modalities such as the CT scan, nuclear scan, MRI, and ultrasonography. With the utilization of plain and contrasted radiographs, patients are being diagnosed earlier with abnormalities and disorders that can now be treated earlier and more definitively. Technological advances will surely lead to more enhanced testing modalities and better and safer testing modalities in the future.

There are many benefits to radiographs such as cost, ease of ordering, and ease of interpretation, as well as utilization of contrasted studies. However, the clarity and definition gained through other radiologic testing such as CT and MRI have led to a decreased use of contrasted radiographs, for example, barium enema. Radiographs are limited by single views and limited contrasting of structures that are overcome with the use of cross-sectional imaging of the body with CT, MRI, and ultrasonography, which will be discussed in this chapter and Chapter 3.

COMPUTED TOMOGRAPHY (CT)

Computed tomography (CT), also known as computed axial tomography (CAT) scanning, was first introduced by Sir Godfrey Hounsfield and Dr. Allan Cormack around 1974. Radiographs produce only one image of one two-dimensional plain from one beam. However, CT scans can produce multiple slices, allowing for reproducible images in three-dimensional plains.

CT scanners employ an x-ray beam that rotates along a circular pattern with detectors rotating along the opposite side. This allows for the system to move in a 360° circle with a well collimated or restricted beam. The beam only travels in one direction through the patient to the detector on the opposite side (Figure 2.4). A complex computer system utilizes algorithms and mathematical formulas to process the data into a large number of two-dimensional slices, like images that can then be formatted into multiple reconstructed plains. The data analyzed by the computer system then assign Hounsfield units (HU) to reconstruct the image based on geometrical plots.

Beam

Motorized table

FIGURE 2.4 CT scanner showing 360° of circle detectors and beams.
Drawing by Ocean City High School student.

Images are composed of a matrix of thousands of tiny squares called pixels. The pixels have a computer-assigned number that correlates to an HU. As discussed earlier, this scale is what produces the shades of gray from black to white. HUs are not absolute and may vary from one CT system to another. HU range from −1,000 to +1,000. However, they can also range from −1,024 to +3,000 or 4,000.

During a CT scan, the patient is placed on a table and the x-ray beam and detector system move through the 360° around them. The detectors receive the x-rays and measure the amount of absorption of the rays as they pass through the body. This data is obtained by the computer and then analyzed and assigned a HU. The computer then produces an image based on the geometric plots of pixels (which are based on the absorption and scatter of the x-ray), resulting in an image on the screen. When viewing the results, the appearance of the images is dependent on the window and level used to display the image. The window describes the range of HUs displayed, and the level describes the center of the window. The wider (or larger) the window, the more types of densities that will be displayed; however, the difference between similar types of tissue lessens, making tissue differentiation difficult to discriminate. The level and window is displayed on every CT image.

The CT image is made up of multiple individual boxes, called pixels. The CT pixel number is proportional to the differences in attenuation of the x-ray by the tissue and is compared with water. The number of pixels can be changed, but they are typically in a matrix (such as 256 × 256). Each image will also have a slice thickness, and the two-dimensional slice will represent all the densities within the volume. The volume of tissue represented by the pixel is called a voxel. The forecastle allows for reconstruction of images by the computer system without losing resolution of the image. Voxel dimensions are determined by the computer system utilizing algorithms that are chosen for the type of reconstruction and are based on the thickness of the scanned slices. If a particular tissue, organ, or lesion is of increased density, then there will be increased absorption, resulting in increased attenuation of the x-ray beam. The more a substance attenuates the beam, the more radiopaque or radiodense it is said to be. On the black and white scale of images on a CT, typically the more radiodense an object is, the closer to white it is displayed. If the particular objects are of decreased density, then there will be decreased absorption of the ray or decreased attenuation, causing a black appearance on the image that is known as radiolucency. You may hear of objects described this way, with a radiodense objection being called a "high density" object (such as a stone or calcification) or "low density" object (such as gas or fat).

The axial view is the traditional view obtained by the computed axial tomography scanner. With the ability to reconstruct images, the computer system can include sagittal, coronal, and oblique plains (Figure 2.5). CT computer systems also utilize volumetric data to produce a three-dimensional image during the reconstruction process (Figure 2.6). This is due to the

(A)

(B)

(C)

FIGURE 2.5 Axial view CT scan (A); sagittal view CT scan (B); and coronal view CT scan (C). Courtesy of Dr. David Begleiter.

ability to produce volumetric data sets. Three-dimensional reconstruction is because of the higher speed scanning of multislice CT and increased computer processing speed and ability.

Conventional single slice scanners were much slower than the technology utilized today with helical or spiral scanners. This is because the patient would hold his or her breath while a single slice was taken and then release his or her breath. The table would then move and this would be repeated. This produced images in slices or sections.

Currently, helical or spiral scanners are utilized to acquire images. These systems allow the table to move at a constant speed, which allows for a more rapid study. Modern systems also include multidetectors, allowing for data to be acquired using rows of detectors that rotate at one time. Multidetector and multislice systems and technology allow for additional

FIGURE 2.6 Three-dimensional CT image.
Courtesy of Dr. David Begleiter.

studies to be derived from the data obtained in one study. An advantage of current CT scanners is their ability for rapid scan acquisition. This rapid scanning allows for larger areas to be scanned in less time with greater resolution. That means that breathing and motion artifacts are greatly reduced; there is greater resolution of images, allowing smaller and smaller objects to be visualized and even allowing scanning of certain areas, such as the coronary arteries, which were never before possible. They also allow for accurate multiplain and three-dimensional reconstruction (this is true of any CT, single or multislice).

CT fluoroscopy can be used with current CT scanners (another advantage of multislice CT). Fluoroscopy improves the performance of image-guided procedures such as biopsies, drainage, and other interventional procedures and is of particular use in guiding needle placement in the chest and abdomen areas that are prone to movement. These CT scans may also be enhanced with the use of contrast, either intravenous, oral, or rectal. Oral and rectal routes are beneficial in visualizing and identifying the bowel and its abnormalities. Intravenous contrast is helpful in enhancing vascular anatomy, vessel patency, and identification of lesions or masses and improves the ability to characterize them. Enhancement assists in differentiating normal anatomy from pathology.

As with radiographs, CT images can be affected by many factors. Artifact has the greatest impact on the clarity of an image. There are many types of artifacts that can affect image quality. If a patient voluntarily or involuntarily moves during the study, it can affect the image, causing prominent streaks from higher to lower density that appear as blurring or shadowing of structures. Metal objects such as surgical clips, staples, and dental fillings can cause streak artifacts because the computer systems are not able to distinguish between high-density sharp-edged objects and adjoining lower density structures. Beam hardening artifacts may be seen as areas of streaking on images, whereas ring artifacts can demonstrate high- or low-density circular rings on the image (Figure 2.7).

(A)

(B)

(C)

(D)

FIGURE 2.7 (A) through (D) demonstrate positron (positive electron) emission tomography scan images.
Courtesy of Dr. David Begleiter.

CT scans are extremely beneficial in diagnosing critical abnormalities and producing real-time images. This allows for CT-guided procedures and fluoroscopy because of the rapid obtaining of images with multislice and multidetector scanners. With the advancements in technology, computer systems allow providers to view areas of interest in multiple plains, including three-dimensional images.

NUCLEAR SCANNING

Nuclear medicine scans and their images are both diagnostic and therapeutic. Nuclear imaging for diagnostic purposes involves a radioactive isotope, an unstable form of an element that emits radiation from its nucleus as it decays, resulting in a stable, but nonradioactive product. Radioactive isotopes occur naturally and artificially. Uranium and thorium are examples of naturally occurring radioactive isotopes. Artificial radioactive isotopes can occur through either neutron enrichment in a nuclear reactor or within a cyclotron. Radioactive isotopes are low dose, nontoxic, and have a short half-life. They are readily incorporated into physiologic compounds and are relatively inexpensive. Technetium 99 m is the most widely used radioisotope in imaging studies.

Radioisotopes are combined and attached to inert agents with binding properties, allowing for concentration in body tissues. Various tissues and organs absorb substances differently. For example, the thyroid best absorbs iodine, the brain best absorbs glucose, and bones best absorb phosphate. Radiopharmaceuticals are referred to as radionuclides, radio tracers, or simply tracers. Most are carried to tissues or organs by the bloodstream; the gamma camera imaging is used to measure radioactive emission. Some agents may be given orally or inhaled, as in ventilation/perfusion (V/Q) scans, or instilled in the bladder for reflux studies. In its simplest form, the gamma camera records radiation emissions from a patient in a single view or plain at point; in its more advanced form, the gamma camera rotates around the patient, acquiring several two-dimensional images from multiple angles. The two-dimensional images are then reconstructed into a three-dimensional data set by a computer. This is known as single-photon emission computed tomography (SPECT).

Positron (positive electron) emission tomography (PET) produces a three-dimensional image depicting the body's biochemistry and metabolic processes at a molecular level. The positive electron or positron radioisotope is attached to a pharmaceutical used in the body's metabolism. This radiopharmaceutical is taken up proportionally with how metabolically active the tissue is. This technique is useful in diagnosing cancer; it is also useful following changes resulting from therapeutic interventions, creating the ability to identify hidden metastasis and recurrence. The PET cyclotron, or generator, produces isotopes with a relatively short half-life that emit positrons. Positrons are significantly higher energy particles that are recorded and used to produce PET images. In general, positron emission generates far less radiation exposure than CT scans or fluoroscopy. However, cardiac PET scanning is known to generate the greatest amount of radiation exposure among all nuclear studies. Figure 2.8 shows examples of PET scan images.

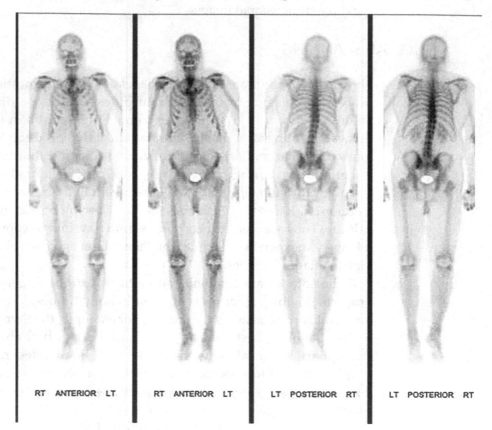

| RT ANTERIOR LT | RT ANTERIOR LT | LT POSTERIOR RT | LT POSTERIOR RT |

FIGURE 2.8 Static image bone scans.
Courtesy of Dr. David Begleiter.

As stated earlier, the half-life is generally shorter with radioisotopes than with other agents. Generally, there are three ways to describe the half-life of a radioisotope. The physical half-life is the period in which an element would decay naturally on its own whether it is sitting on the shelf in a container or if it has been administered; that is, the time at which half of the original radioactivity is gone. The biologic half-life is based on the normal physiologic removal of the radioisotope and the pharmaceutical. For example, when it is excreted from the kidneys and/or the gastrointestinal tract, the biologic half-life is shorter than the natural physical half-life. Finally, effective half-life is a mathematical derivation based on formulas that combine biologic and physical parameters. It is a measurement of when the actual isotope remains effective within the body.

PET scanning can be used in conjunction with a CT scan to give a more accurate localization of an abnormality or lesion for surgery or biopsy, or to identify suspected metastasis. When PET and SPECT CT scanning are performed together, there is an increased specificity and sensitivity in the cardiac, neural, and oncological identification of abnormalities. These enhanced imaging modalities also improve the identification of malignancies and staging of treatment in cancer patients.

Nuclear imaging is unique in its ability to provide high functional resolution, providing physiologic as well as functional information of organ structure that is not otherwise available with CT, MRI, or ultrasound imaging. Functional imaging identifies whether an organ is normally or abnormally functioning, independent from anatomical abnormalities.

Two types of images can be obtained with a nuclear study: static or dynamic. Static images evaluate organs and areas in a still state, such as thyroid scans, liver scans, splenic scans, and so on (Figure 2.9). Dynamic images include rapid sequence images of moving areas such as blood flow to organs, muscles of the skeleton, and renal perfusion. Nuclear imaging is based on the detection and mapping of the biodistribution of radio tracers that have been administered and captured by emission imaging. Table 2.1 demonstrates the five

TABLE 2.1 The Five Basic Isotope Concentrations in the Body

Type of Isotope Concentration	Scan	Absorption	Evaluates
Blood pool or compartment localization	Cardiac	Glucose	Perfusion
			Function
			Viability
	Brain		Mass
Physiological inclusion	Thyroid	Iodine	Goiter
			Hyperthyroid
			Cancer
	Bone	Phosphates	Metastasis
			Abuse
Capillary blockage	Lung		Pulmonary embolus (obstruction)
			Quantitative perfusion
Phagocytosis	Liver		Cholestasis
			Mass
			Metastasis
Cell sequestration	Spleen		Injury
			Mass

(A)

(B)

FIGURE 2.9 Dynamic image; pre-exercise nuclear stress test (A); large antero apical and septal ischemia (B). Note loss of areas in all three views compared to a normal scan. Courtesy of Dr. Yatish B. Merchant.

basic isotope concentrations in the body, the mechanism, the type of study, what is assessed in that study, and what is absorbed by that particular organ with consideration of radioisotopes attaching to pharmaceuticals.

Nuclear imaging allows for identification of abnormal tissue, such as cancer and metastasis, and provides imaging, reflecting the functionality of an organ and/or system. Innovations in the field of nuclear imaging include molecular medicine and molecular imaging, applying genomics and protein messaging that allows the following of gene therapy as well as stem cell therapy from its introduction into the patient. The capabilities of nuclear imaging allow the diagnosis of abnormalities and can measure therapeutic effects so interventions can be modified based on the patient's response.

CONCLUSION

The three radiating testing modalities are similar in the foundation of how the image is obtained. However, CT and nuclear imaging take this foundation further with multiple views, contrast, and digital technology. When deciding on the appropriate testing modality to order, it is important to take into consideration how the images are obtained and what you are looking to achieve.

Consideration must be taken into account for the amount of radiation exposure a patient receives from every radiological study. The risk and benefit as well as the necessity of each study must be weighed carefully to protect patients. A radiation dose of 50 millisieverts (mSv) can place a person at risk for cancer. A CT of the abdomen and pelvis can emit approximately 30 mSv when performed with and without contrast. Correlation of cancer to radiation exposure can take one to two decades, making it difficult to determine the actual risk.

RESOURCES

American College of Radiology. (n.d.). Appropriateness criteria. Retrieved from http://www.acr.org/quality-safety/appropriateness-criteria

Au-Yong, I., Au-Yong, A., & Broderick, N. (2010). *On-call x-rays made easy.* Philadelphia, PA: Churchill Livingstone, Elsevier.

Badawi, R. D., Kroger, L. A., & Bushberg, J. T. (2012). Essential science of nuclear medicine. In W. E. Brant & C. A. Helms (Eds.), *Fundamentals of diagnostic radiology* (4th ed., pp. 1233–1249). Philadelphia, PA: Wolters Kluwer/Lippincott Williams & Wilkins.

Brant, W. E. (2012). Diagnostic imaging methods. In W. E. Brant & C. A. Helms (Eds.), *Fundamentals of diagnostic radiology* (4th ed., pp. 2–27). Philadelphia, PA: Wolters Kluwer/Lippincott Williams & Wilkins.

Cameron, C. F., Bijan, B., & Shelton, D. K. (2012). Positron emission tomography. In W. E. Brant & C. A. Helms (Eds.), *Fundamentals of diagnostic radiology* (4th ed., pp. 1388–1419). Philadelphia, PA: Wolters Kluwer/Lippincott Williams & Wilkins.

Daffner, R. H. (2014). Overview and principles of diagnostic imaging. In R. H. Daffner & M. S. Hartman (Eds.), *Clinical radiology: The essentials* (4th ed., pp. 1–42). Philadelphia, PA: Wolters Kluwer/Lippincott Williams & Wilkins.

Daffner, R. H., & Hartman, R. H. (2014). Radiographic contrast agents. In R. H. Daffner & M. S. Hartman (Eds.), *Clinical radiology: The essentials* (4th ed., pp. 43–48). Philadelphia, PA: Wolters Kluwer/Lippincott Williams & Wilkins.

Donnelly, L. F. (2009). *Pediatric imaging: The fundamentals*. Philadelphia, PA: Saunders Elsevier.

Herring, W. (2016). *Learning radiology: Recognizing the basics* (3rd ed., pp. 1–7). Philadelphia, PA: Elsevier.

Shelton, D. K. (2012). Introduction to nuclear medicine. In W. E. Brant & C. A. Helms, *Fundamentals of diagnostic radiology* (4th ed., pp. 1228–1232). Philadelphia, PA: Wolters Kluwer/Lippincott Williams & Wilkins.

Nonradiating Testing Modalities

This chapter introduces and briefly discusses the two testing modalities that do not use ionizing radiation to produce an image. Each testing modality is described, including how the images are obtained by the various machines and technology, their uses and benefits, and limitations. This allows for differentiating the various modalities and provides an appreciation for how the images are produced. Understanding the various testing modalities is fundamental in deciding what tests are most useful for diagnostic purposes.

MAGNETIC RESONANCE IMAGING (MRI)

MRI was simultaneously discovered by two physicists, Felix Bloch and Edward Mills Purcell, in the late 1940s; both men won the Nobel Prize in 1952 for their discovery. However, it was not until the late 1970s when Paul Lauterbur, Peter Mansfield, and Raymond Damadian began using MRIs and clinical images in the diagnostic study of patients.

The science behind MRI is quite different from that of radiographs and CT scans. MRI does not use ionizing radiation for the development of images but rather uses the inherent magnetism of tissues, especially hydrogen in water, which constitutes approximately 70% of the human body. MRI scanners use very strong magnetic fields and radiofrequency waves to manipulate the electromagnetic activity of protons within the hydrogen nucleus. The radiofrequency waves influence the spin of the protons used to produce the image, changing the magnetic fields. The energy released in this process is then received by coils in the scanner and processed by a computer to form an image (Figure 3.1).

FIGURE 3.1 MR image.
Courtesy of Dr. David Begleiter.

An MRI machine consists of the primary magnet, gradient magnet, gradient coils, radiofrequency coils, radiofrequency detector, and a computer. The human body consists primarily of water (70%), which is comprised of two hydrogen and one oxygen atom held together by magnetic bonds. Each hydrogen atom has a single spinning proton; a charged proton particle produces a magnetic field referred to as a magnetic moment (Figure 3.2A). These hydrogen protons are randomly oriented until a very strong magnet is applied. The magnetic force utilized to make up the primary magnetic field in an MRI is 50,000 times stronger than the magnetic field of the Earth. When the primary magnetic field is turned on, it causes hydrogen protons to spin on an axis parallel to the magnet, like a spinning top (Figure 3.2B). Radiofrequency coils within the MRI transmit short radio frequency waves or pulses that change the orientation of the protons. When the radiofrequency pulse is turned off or stops, it allows the proton to relax and return to its prior state of alignment with the primary magnetic field. When this occurs, energy is released in the form of radiofrequency signals; these are then read by the receiving radiofrequency coils. Gradient magnet and gradient coils all have areas of varying magnetic strength, which aid in the reading of energy exerted by the proton when applied with the radiofrequency waves. The radiofrequency coils send their received information to the radiofrequency detector; this is ultimately entered into a computer along with the information received from the gradient coils, which input the received information directly into the computer. An image is the final production (Figure 3.3).

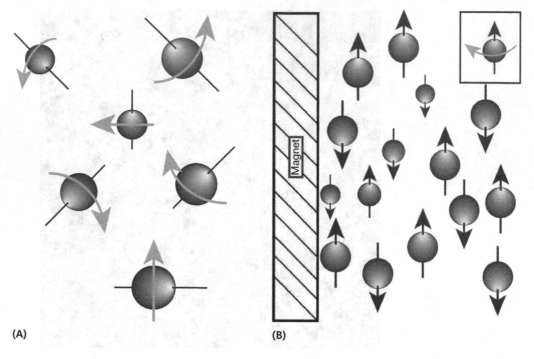

FIGURE 3.2 Hydrogen atoms spinning in different directions (A) and hydrogen atoms lined up with magnet (B).
Drawing by Ocean City High School student.

FIGURE 3.3 MR scanner labeled by parts.
Drawing by Ocean City High School student.

When reviewing an MR image, the energy produced by changes in the magnetic charge within body tissues is transformed by the computer into images that depict the tissue type. If tissue has little to no hydrogen, such as cortical bone or air within the lung, a dark or black area will appear on the image (Figure 3.4). Conversely, if the tissue is high in hydrogen, such as occurs in the brain, spinal column, heart, abdominal viscera and organs, and musculoskeletal system, a white area will appear on the image (Figure 3.5). For this reason, MR imaging is best for identifying abnormalities within these structures. MR angiography is also useful in identifying vascular abnormalities in assessing organ function. Functional MRI studies of the brain, for example, can be interpreted through changes in blood perfusion to tissue regions as seen through captured images.

FIGURE 3.4 Little amount of hydrogen in tissue. Courtesy of Dr. David Begleiter; diagramming, Theresa M. Campo.

FIGURE 3.5 Large amount of hydrogen in tissue. Courtesy of Dr. David Begleiter; diagramming, Theresa M. Campo.

MRI has many uses, as discussed, and is considered to be safe during pregnancy since no ionizing radiation is used; therefore, it can detect suspected cholecystitis and appendicitis, which are common during pregnancy. Since strong magnets are used during the imaging process, patients must be screened prior to imaging for any implanted metallic substances, such as pacemakers or artificial valves or joints, to avoid displacement or complications. It is also important to ascertain if patients have any known or potential retained metallic foreign bodies, especially in the eyes, brain, or other vital areas of the body that may move or shift, causing adverse complications during the study. Since MRI studies require patients to remain still within an enclosed space for prolonged durations, it is important to assess for claustrophobia and anxiety since motion artifacts can result in an inadequate image or imaging series due to the sensitivity of the recall coils receiving information at the atomic level. Patients prone to anxiety or claustrophobia may need to be medicated prior to the test or scanned with an open MRI scanner. However, open scanners may result in poorer quality images because their magnetic strength is decreased.

Since its development and use in the 1970s, MRI has allowed for more precise and detailed imaging of the body, and is safer in that it does not utilize ionizing radiation to produce an image. As with radiographs and CT scans, contrast MRI imaging can assist in identifying different types of tissues and organs. MRI is very sensitive in differentiating soft tissue structures such as ligaments, tendons, and muscle. Because the technology uses very strong magnets, care must be given in screening patients for surgical clips, body piercings, pacemakers, and other metallic apparatus. Additionally, it is important to consider the location of objects within the external environment, such as oxygen tanks and intravenous poles, and so forth. MRI technology is also useful in generating detailed three-dimensional images.

ULTRASONOGRAPHY

Ultrasonography, also known as ultrasound, has been around since its development and first use in the 1940s. Ultrasound uses sound waves to generate real-time images. Ultrasound is a noninvasive method to evaluate anatomical structures and function and is also used for guiding and increasing accuracy in performing invasive procedures, such as joint aspiration and intravenous catheter insertion. Ultrasound can be performed at the bedside as well as in the radiology department or outpatient setting.

Ultrasound uses sound waves or pulses at a range of 1 to 17 MHz, which is well above the human's ability to hear sound—between 20 and 20,000 Hz. The ultrasound probe or transducer both sends out and receives sound waves that are then interpreted by a computer, which generates an image in real time. The transducer transmits extremely short bursts of sound waves that are able to penetrate tissue. Once the sound waves reach the interface of the tissue, they return to the transducer as an echo; this echo is interpreted into an image based on the round-trip time of the pulse and echo. Once the echo arrives back to the transducer, it is converted to electrical pulses that are sent to the scanner and computer, generating an image. Figure 3.6 demonstrates how ultrasonography works.

The final image is created by the difference between the amount of sound that is transmitted from the transducer compared with that reflected back through the echo. If sound waves encounter a fluid-filled structure, most of the energy will be transmitted and appear as well-defined walls. While this may be an indication of a cyst, it is not due to the fluid nature of the cyst but rather the decreased reflection of sound or an absence of internal echo, which appears dark or black on the image. This is commonly referred to as being

To signal processor

Source

Detector

Ultrasound gel

Subject

FIGURE 3.6 How ultrasonography works.
Drawing by Ocean City High School student.

hypoechoic (Figure 3.7). If these sound waves encounter bone or air, most of the energy is either deflected or absorbed and is seen as a bright or white shading on the image, referred to as hyperechoic (Figure 3.8). As with other testing modalities, there are shades and patterns between the spectrums of white and black. For example, solid tissue may have a speckled appearance with definable, visible blood vessels that appear lighter because of the hyperechoic property of vessel walls. Conversely, solid organs and fluid, which are hypoechoic, will appear darker.

Ultrasonography is performed with a patient in a comfortable position with the transducer placed on the skin against the area to be imaged. A coupling agent, consisting of a water-soluble gel or other media, is applied to the transducer to ensure good contact and transmission of the ultrasonic waves in a controlled manner through the skin to the underlying structures. As stated earlier, transducers have the ability to produce high-frequency sound waves between 1 and 17 MHz. Higher frequency

FIGURE 3.7 Fluid-filled area—hypoechoic.
Source: Theresa M. Campo/ Aubrey Rybinski.

FIGURE 3.8 Air or bone—hyperechoic.
Source: Theresa M. Campo/ Aubrey Rybinski.

waves produce clearer images than lower frequencies and result in less tissue penetration, making them more useful when imaging superficial structures, such as the thyroid or breasts, or when imaging infants and small children. Conversely, lower frequency waves have good tissue penetration and are best for evaluating deeper structures, such as those within the abdomen or the pelvis. However, these images lose some of their resolution.

Ultrasound images can be produced in various anatomical plains such as the axial, coronal, or sagittal plains based on the position of the transducer with regard to the position of the patient or area being studied. Transducers can also be placed inside the body, such as transvaginal, transesophageal, transrectal, or intraoral transducers, for better visualization of deep or difficult-to-see organs or structures. Since sonic waves do not readily penetrate bone or gas-filled areas, acoustic windows are used to visualize underlying structures. For example, evaluation of the liver is performed through acoustic windows in the intercostal spaces of the ribs. A transabdominal ultrasound uses the bladder to better visualize and block the air-filled colon. There are five types of ultrasound as seen in Table 3.1.

TABLE 3.1 Types of Ultrasound

Mode	Information
A-mode (amplitude mode)	• Simplest type • Single transducer • Spikes along a line represent the amplitude of the signal at different depths • Therapeutic scan is also done in this mode to treat tumors or calculi
B-mode (brightness mode)	• Most often used • Also known as two-dimensional • Each echo is depicted as a dot, with thousands of dots making an image
M-mode (motion mode)	• Quick pulses in quick succession • Evaluate moving structures
Doppler	• Determines flow and velocity of blood • Shows on monitor screen as blue or red • Red Indicates flow toward the transducer • Blue indicates flow away from the transducer
Duplex	• Simultaneously uses gray-scale and color Doppler to visualize flow within the vessel

Ultrasound has numerous benefits, which are increasing with advancing technology. Ultrasound provides static and dynamic real-time images, is used to increase accuracy when performing procedures, is safe to use during pregnancy and with children, and is less expensive than other testing modalities such as MRI and CT scanning. Limitations include difficulty in crossing tissue–gas and tissue–bone interfaces; in addition, image quality and interpretation are operator dependent. Therefore, it is vital that the ultrasound user become proficient in ultrasound technique for diagnostic and therapeutic purposes.

CONSIDERATIONS WHEN ORDERING DIAGNOSTIC MEDICAL IMAGING

When deciding on the most appropriate imaging modality to order, it is important to take into consideration how the images are obtained and what you are looking to achieve with the diagnosis. Diagnostic imaging does not replace taking a thorough history and performing a physical examination.

The decision to add an imaging study must include consideration of risks and benefits, cost to the patient as well as to the institution, and potential adverse effects (i.e., anaphylaxis, teratogenic harm during pregnancy). Collaboration with colleagues, including radiologists and radiology technologists, is key to achieving appropriate care of the patient and identification of problems or potential problems.

Resources to improve decision making in diagnostic imaging include use of the American College of Radiology (ACR) Appropriateness Criteria, which are evidence-based and regularly updated. These guidelines and algorithms are organized by symptom and suspected condition and aid in decision making.

The ACR Appropriateness Criteria provide quality ratings for various medical imaging studies based on complaint or working diagnosis. For example, if a pulmonary embolus is suspected, a list of radiological studies is listed with ratings, comments, and the relative radiation level. Rating scales range from 1 to 9, with 1 to 3 being "usually not appropriate," 4 to 6 "may be appropriate," and 7 to 9 "usually appropriate."

CONCLUSION

MRI and ultrasound, although different in how they produce physical images, are similar in safety since neither involves exposure to ionizing radiation. MRI has many advantages, including the contrast of images and the ability to reconstruct images for enhanced detail. Disadvantages include cost, time to complete the study, and potential complications from implanted metallic medical devices. In addition, some patients may not be able to tolerate the restrictions imposed during testing.

The benefits of ultrasound include cost, safety, portable access, and real-time imaging, making diagnosis and therapeutic interventions much easier. Limitations include image quality that is highly operator dependent and difficult to obtain in the morbidly obese individual or when imagining structures through bone and air/gas. However, its use is increasing with smaller, more digitally enhanced machines.

RESOURCES

American College of Radiology. (n.d.). Appropriateness criteria. Retrieved from http://www.acr.org/quality-safety/appropriateness-criteria

Au-Yong, I., Au-Yong, A., & Broderick, N. (2010). *On-call x-rays made easy*. Philadelphia, PA: Churchill Livingstone, Elsevier.

Brant, W. E. (2012). Abdomen ultrasound. In W. E. Brant & C. A. Helms (Eds.), *Fundamentals of diagnostic radiology* (4th ed., pp. 858–885). Philadelphia, PA: Wolters Kluwer/Lippincott Williams & Wilkins.

Brant, W. E. (2012). Chest, thyroid, parathyroid, and neonatal brain. In W. E. Brant & C. A. Helms (Eds.), *Fundamentals of diagnostic radiology* (4th ed., pp. 936–953). Philadelphia, PA: Wolters Kluwer/Lippincott Williams & Wilkins.

Brant, W. E. (2012). Diagnostic imaging methods. In W. E. Brant & C. A. Helms (Eds.), *Fundamentals of diagnostic radiology* (4th ed., pp. 2–27). Philadelphia, PA: Wolters Kluwer/Lippincott Williams & Wilkins.

Brant, W. E. (2012). Genital tract and bladder ultrasound. In W. E. Brant & C. A. Helms (Eds.), *Fundamentals of diagnostic radiology* (4th ed., pp. 886–909). Philadelphia, PA: Wolters Kluwer/Lippincott Williams & Wilkins.

Brant, W. E., & Dougherty, R. S. (2012). Vascular ultrasound. In W. E. Brant & C. A. Helms (Eds.), *Fundamentals of diagnostic radiology* (4th ed., pp. 954–979). Philadelphia, PA: Wolters Kluwer/Lippincott Williams & Wilkins.

Daffner, R. H. (2014). Overview and principles of diagnostic imaging. In R. H. Daffner & M. S. Hartman (Eds.), *Clinical radiology: The essentials* (4th ed., pp. 1–42). Philadelphia, PA: Wolters Kluwer/Lippincott Williams & Wilkins.

Daffner, R. H., & Hartman, R. H. (2014). Radiographic contrast agents. In R. H. Daffner & M. S. Hartman (Eds.), *Clinical radiology: The essentials* (4th ed., pp. 43–48). Philadelphia, PA: Wolters Kluwer/Lippincott Williams & Wilkins.

Herring, W. (2016). *Learning radiology: Recognizing the basics* (3rd ed., pp. 1–7, 204–227) Philadelphia, PA: Elsevier.

Interpreting Chest and Abdominal Radiographs

Basic Interpretation of the Chest

The interpretation of chest radiographs can be gratifying as well as frustrating. It can take many years of experience looking at radiographs to gain competency and confidence in interpretation. However, we all have to start somewhere, so this chapter is meant to introduce you to the basic interpretation of chest radiographs. This chapter includes a brief review of the radiographic densities discussed earlier in this book, adequacy of radiographs and why this is important, and pediatric considerations. It is important to understand what you're looking at so you can identify not only normal structures but also abnormal findings. Plain radiographs are excellent in evaluating normal structures of the chest, foreign bodies, and gross abnormalities within the chest and surrounding structures that may lead to further radiological evaluation.

RADIOGRAPHIC DENSITIES

Radiographic density refers to the degree of blackness of the film. It allows for radiographic contrast, and therefore provides the ability to differentiate various structures (Figure 4.1). Structures with high physical density produce less radiodensity and vice versa. When a structure has a low radiodensity, the rays easily penetrate the structure, resulting in low absorbency; this causes blackening of the film. When a structure has a high radiodensity, the passage of rays is impeded; in other words, there is high absorbency; this results in a bright or white appearance on the film. Structures with varying degrees of radiodensity and absorption or attenuation will give varying shades of gray between the spectrum of black and white. Contrast between adjacent structures is increased when there is a difference in radiodensity or thickness of those structures. Whether evaluating the structures of the chest, abdomen, spine, or extremities, this spectrum is important in understanding exactly what you are visualizing on the radiographs. Figure 4.1 demonstrates these concepts.

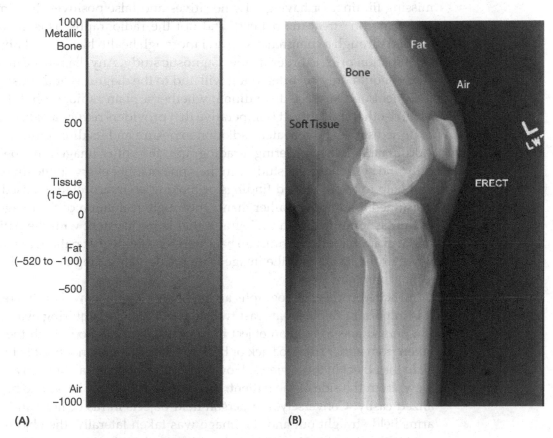

FIGURE 4.1 Radiographic density (A) and radiographic contrast of structures (B).
Drawing by Ocean City High School student (A). Courtesy of Dr. David Begleiter; diagramming, Theresa M. Campo (B).

ADEQUACY OF RADIOGRAPHS

Image quality is paramount to being able to accurately review and identify normal and abnormal findings on radiographs. Image quality can be affected by motion, scatter, magnification, thickness, and distortion, as discussed in Chapter 2 of this text. When reviewing radiographs, one must remember that the body is three-dimensional; however, radiographs produce two-dimensional images through shades of gray, which depict structures of varying densities. It is also important to have a firm recollection and understanding of basic anatomy and physiology. When discussing, reporting, and documenting findings of the chest x-ray, it is important to remember that these are findings and not diagnoses. Stating that you visualize a patchy infiltrate of the right middle lobe is a finding. However, stating that you visualize a right middle lobe pneumonia is not correct because a diagnosis results from a synthesis of a thorough health history and physical examination findings, along with the finding of a patchy infiltrate in the right middle lobe.

As with anything in medicine and nursing, there are rules in place to help not only guide the interpretation of radiographs, but also to help avoid missing findings or having false negatives and false positives. It is important that you "treat the patient" and not the radiographs. This is accomplished through a comprehensive and thorough health history and physical examination prior to ordering the diagnostic study. Any diagnostic imaging study should only be ordered if it will add to the diagnosis and subsequent treatment of a suspected condition, whether a plain radiograph, CT scan, MRI, or other modality. It is imperative that providers reduce a patient's risk of unnecessary and repeated radiation exposure and its dire consequences. Additionally, when ordering a radiograph, the entire image must be carefully and systematically studied in the same manner every single time. This will help to avoid missed findings or making an interpretation based on a presumed assumption rather than a thorough evaluation of the image. If a finding is identified on a radiograph that is inconsistent with the patient's initial examination, one must go back and reevaluate that patient to identify whether the finding on the image is an incidental finding or related to the initial complaint.

As stated earlier, radiographs are taken in a single view. For this reason, it is important to obtain at least two views of an area requiring evaluation. If a person was to hold an object in front of his or her body with the x-ray taken from either front to back or back to front, one may not be able to visualize the object in those views. However, if the image is taken from a lateral view, from the side of the patient, then the object would be able to be visualized easily. Conversely, if a person held objects in his or her hands with arms held straight out and the image was taken laterally, the objects may not be readily seen. However, an anterior or posterior view would provide an image of the laterally held objects. It is also important to compare current with previous studies to ascertain changes over time as well as to confirm normal anatomy for that particular individual. When evaluating extremities, comparison views can be very helpful, especially in pediatric patients, to identify if a finding is abnormal or normal. To ensure quality and safety in diagnostic interpretation, all radiographs should be reviewed by experienced and trained radiologists in addition to the provider who is evaluating the patient. Continued collaboration with radiologists and radiology technicians, as well as colleagues, is imperative for quality care of all patients.

Before interpretation of a chest x-ray can begin, confirming the patient's name, date, and correct study must be assessed. Once confirmation is complete, then determination of adequacy of the film must be done. Position, inspiration, penetration, and rotation need to be considered in order to deem a study to be adequate. The direction that the beam travels through the patient and the cassette determines the title of the position. When the patient is facing the cartridge with the x-ray machine behind him or her, the image is labeled posterior–anterior (PA); conversely, if the cartridge is behind the patient with the machine in front of him or her, the image is labeled anterior–posterior (AP) (Figure 4.2). The PA view is most often performed for optimal evaluation of the chest. The heart and mediastinum sit more anteriorly in the chest; when imaged in this view, they are more true to size. The AP view is usually done as a portable image. When the rays travel from the front to the back of the person, magnification occurs; this causes the heart and mediastinum to appear bigger in size and not as clear as they truly are.

(A)   (B)

FIGURE 4.2 Posterior–anterior (A) versus anterior–posterior view (B). Note the hazy borders and markings, large heart, widened aorta, and white appearance of the film, overall.
Courtesy of Dr. David Begleiter.

A lateral view image is when the patient is standing between the cassette and the x-ray machine and the beam is traveling right to left (Figure 4.3). The lateral decubitus view image requires that the patient lie on his or her side for 3 to 5 minutes before the frontal view is taken. This allows for any fluid to settle and air to rise, which may demonstrate free air or fluid abnormalities (Figure 4.4). All films should be marked left or right along with the view. For example, if an AP view is taken and not labeled, it may be assumed that it is a PA view, leading to a false reading that results from normal differences of the two views. In a normal PA view, the lung markings are more distinct, the heart is smaller, the clavicles are superimposed over the upper lung fields, and the cervical and thoracic vertebrae are more clearly visible (Figure 4.5). However, in the AP view, the heart appears larger than normal with shallow long volumes and higher sitting clavicles (Figure 4.6).

FIGURE 4.3 Lateral view.

FIGURE 4.4 Lateral decubitus view.

FIGURE 4.5 Posterior–anterior chest.
Courtesy of Dr. David Begleiter.

FIGURE 4.6 Anterior–posterior chest.

During any chest radiographic imaging, the patient will be asked to take a deep breath and hold it. This allows for better visualization of the structures within and around the chest cavity. Normal inspiration is determined by counting the anterior and posterior ribs. The diaphragm should cross the level of the 10th posterior rib; however, as long as it is between the 8th and 10th posterior ribs or at the level of the fifth or sixth anterior ribs, the image is acceptable. One would think that the ribs appearing to be closest to the person viewing the film are the anterior ribs. However, they are actually the posterior ribs (Figure 4.7). If there is a poor inspiratory effort, the film may not be accurately evaluated, as demonstrated in Figure 4.8. A chest radiograph may also be performed during expiration. This method is used to evaluate a patient for either pneumothorax or a foreign body in the bronchus. During expiration, a foreign body in the bronchus may cause a shift in the mediastinum and heart due to the lack of volume in the affected side. Similarly, during expiration, you may see enlargement of a pneumothorax, making it more visible.

Differences in physical density impact the penetration and absorption of x-rays. If structures are not properly penetrated, there will be poor film quality with regard to clarity and shifts in the shades of gray spectrum. The same radiation dose cannot be used for all patients since body size will affect ray penetration, which can result in over- or underexposed images negatively affecting the adequacy of the film.

Normally, in the PA view, you should be able to visualize the thoracic spine through the heart shadow and be able to see the intravertebral discs of the upper cervical spine (Figure 4.9). Underpenetration can cause an image to be too light; if this happens, the thoracic spine will not be visible through the heart shadow (Figure 4.10). Additionally, the hemidiaphragm

FIGURE 4.7 Inspiration with proper number of ribs.
Courtesy of Dr. David Begleiter.

FIGURE 4.8 Poor inspiration. Note the height of the diaphragms and distortion of structures.
Courtesy of Dr. David Begleiter.

FIGURE 4.9 Normal chest posterior–anterior view.
Courtesy of Dr. David Begleiter.

may not be visible; consequently, it may be mistaken for a left lower lobe infiltrate, consolidation, or pleural effusion. When an image is overpenetrated, it appears dark with decreased or loss of lung markings that can be mistaken for emphysema or a pneumothorax (Figure 4.11).

Finally, rotation can also have a negative effect on film adequacy. Distortion of normal anatomical structures can occur when a patient is rotated (Figure 4.12). It is important that patients stand as

FIGURE 4.10 Underpenetration.
Courtesy of Dr. David Begleiter.

FIGURE 4.11 Overpenetration.
Courtesy of Dr. Keith Lafferty.

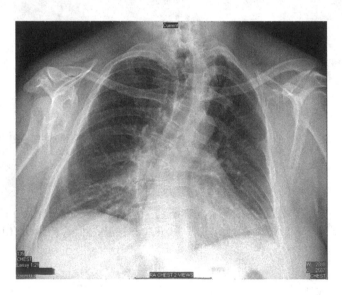

FIGURE 4.12 Rotation.
Courtesy of Dr. David Begleiter.

parallel to the cassette with shoulders back, taking a deep breath and hold-ing it. If the person has one shoulder in front of the other, this can cause rotation and inadequacy of that image. The heads of the clavicle, ribs, and spinal processes should be symmetrical and at equal heights bilaterally. A trick to determining rotation is to look at the medial aspects of the clav-icles in relation to the spinal processes to see that they are of equal height and also appear equally spaced from one side to the other.

Once adequacy has been determined and accepted, then the interpretation of the film can begin. When interpreting any radiographs, it is important to remember the ABCDEs. They are *a*dequacy/*a*irway, *b*reathing or *b*irdcages, *c*ardiac/*c*irculation, *d*iaphragm, *e*dges, and *s*keleton/*s*oft tissue.

We have already discussed the adequacy of the film and now we are going to discuss the other *A*, which is *a*irway. The trachea should be midline and seen to the carina (tracheal bifurcation) at the approximate level of the T4 to T5 interspace (Figure 4.13). These are air-filled tubes, so they should have a dark appearance because they are surrounded by soft tissue, which is lighter in color and allows for contrast. The trachea should angle downward to the thoracic inlet and be identifiable by the retrotracheal line, which should not exceed 3 mm. One is able to visualize the structures because they are surrounded by soft tissue, which appears lighter; this gives the contrasting appearance. If there is thickening of the outlining of the airway, then it is labeled a bronchogram. A bronchogram is made visible by the surrounding alveoli containing fluid or exudate such as mucus. A bronchogram can be diagnostic for neoplasm, severe interstitial disease,

(A)   (B)

FIGURE 4.13 Airway. Please note the darkening of the airway against the lighter wall. In (A) you should visualize the trachea to the carina (bifurcation); in (B) you can also visualize the airway. Courtesy of Dr. David Begleiter; diagramming, Theresa M. Campo.

pulmonary edema, consolidation, or nonobstructive pulmonary atelectasis. However, a bronchogram in some individuals may be normal and not a sign of pathology (Figure 4.14).

(A)

(B)

(C)

FIGURE 4.14 Bronchogram. (A) demonstrates a bronchogram on plain radiograph and (B) and (C) demonstrate a contrasted radiograph.
Courtesy of Associate Professor Frank Gaillard, Radiopaedia.org.

When evaluating the **B** of our ABCs, we think about breathing. I like to evaluate this by looking at the birdcages (Figure 4.15). If you look at the area on each side of the pleural cavity encasing the lungs, they have the appearance of the birdcage. You want to evaluate both birdcages and note whether they are comparable in appearance. You should be able to

FIGURE 4.15 Breathing/birdcages. Courtesy of Dr. David Begleiter; diagramming, Theresa M. Campo.

visualize the pleural tissue filling both birdcages. If you notice a brighter or whiter area in one birdcage that is not in the other, then you need to identify the finding as an abnormality. This is where knowledge of basic anatomy is key in identifying structures within the birdcage and abnormalities.

Each lung lobe has anatomical segments that are supplied by their own bronchus and blood vessels. The right lung has three lobes—the upper, middle, and lower—and the left has two lobes—the upper and lower. The segments of the right upper lobe are the apical, anterior, and posterior segments. The middle lobe includes the medial and lateral segments. The lower lobe has the most segments and includes the superior, posterior, medial, anterior, and lateral base segments. The left upper lobe has a fused apical–posterior segment, as well as anterior, superior, and inferior segments. The left lower lobe is similar to the right lower lobe except the anterior and medial basal segments are fused.

The pleura is made up of two layers: the visceral and parietal layers. The visceral layer covers the lung and is not readily visualized on radiographs. However, it may be normal to visualize the interlobar fissures. There are two interlobar fissures on the right: the oblique, or major, and the horizontal, or minor. The left interlobar fissure consists of only the oblique fissure. The oblique fissures are normally at the level of T4 and extend downward, ending at the anterior sixth rib. The horizontal fissure begins at the level of the sixth rib and then extends laterally and anteriorly downward to the medial section of the fourth rib.

The center of the chest is where we look for our **C**, which represents the cardiac silhouette and circulation (Figure 4.16). You will note that the heart silhouette sits in the center, slightly to the left. At the superior aspect of the heart, you will notice the aorta, which should be small and not enlarged or tortuous. You will also notice the branches of a tree coming out into each of our birdcages, which is the pulmonary vasculature. The heart silhouette should be less than half the width of the chest cavity. One would think that the tracings in the birdcage would be the bronchi, but they are actually the pulmonary vasculature. The bronchi are air filled and hidden by the air in the lungs, which obscures them due to the similar density. One is able to visualize the vasculature because it is fluid filled against the air-filled lungs and bronchi, allowing for contrast and visualization. If the heart silhouette goes beyond the midline, then it is considered to be enlarged. Roughly the cardiothoracic ratio should be 1:2.

FIGURE 4.16 Cardiac/circulation. Courtesy of Dr. David Begleiter; diagramming, Theresa M. Campo.

Our diaphragms represent the **D** of our ABCDEs. The right hemidiaphragm sits higher than the left hemidiaphragm due to the contiguity of the left ventricle of the heart with the left diaphragm. It is not because of the bulk or size of the liver (Figure 4.17). When both diaphragms are sitting at the same level, it can be due to normal physiologic reasons, such as with pregnancy, which can push up the left hemidiaphragm, or from pathologic causes such as diaphragmatic rupture or other trauma. Emphysema can cause blunting of the costophrenic angles at the lateral aspect of the diaphragm because of excessive air trapping.

The **E** is for edges. What you want to do here is look at the edges of your birdcage and its contents to see that the edges are crisp and clearly

(A)

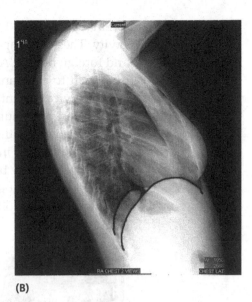
(B)

FIGURE 4.17 Diaphragms on posterior–anterior view (A) and lateral view (B).
Courtesy of Dr. David Begleiter; diagramming, Theresa M. Campo.

visualized (Figure 4.18). If you notice hazing or blurring of any of these edges, it may indicate an abnormality. For example, blurring or hazing indicating an increased density over the right diaphragm may be suggestive of a right lower lobe infiltrate or consolidation.

FIGURE 4.18 Edges.
Courtesy of Dr. David Begleiter; diagramming, Theresa M. Campo.

Finally, we need to evaluate the skeleton and soft tissue outside the chest cavity. These are important areas to evaluate for fractures, neoplasm, free air, and foreign bodies. Again, it is imperative that you evaluate the entire radiograph left to right and top to bottom, including everything in between. The lower cervical (pointing down) and thoracic vertebrae (pointing up), ribs, clavicles, scapula, humeral heads, and the sternum (lateral view only) should all be visualized on the chest radiograph. The radiographs should also include identifiable patient information, the date, and technologist markers, as well as the type of study being done. With the age of digital technology, the identifiable patient demographic information, as well as the type of study, reason for this study, and ordering provider, may be separate from the image itself (Figure 4.19).

FIGURE 4.19 Skeletal/ soft tissue.
Courtesy of Dr. David Begleiter.

ABCs are performed when evaluating radiographs to allow providers to identify normal from abnormal findings. Discussion of the type of abnormal findings that can be visualized on a radiograph is discussed in Chapter 5. The ability to identify what is occurring in a pathologic process will assist in anticipating and visualizing findings on radiographs. For example, pathology of the air spaces may be identified as consolidation or atelectasis because the normally air-filled areas are either fluid filled or the walls have collapsed. Fluid accumulation in the pleural space is identified as an effusion, emphysema and asthma may result from over-inflation of the lungs, and interstitial changes may be from fibrosis and/ or edema. Over time, with practice in viewing multiple chest radiographs, differentiating normal from abnormal findings will only get easier and you will begin to feel more confident reviewing and documenting findings. I guarantee you'll enjoy the process as you get more proficient and comfortable with your interpretations.

PEDIATRIC CONSIDERATIONS (COMPARISON OF ADULT AND INFANT/CHILD)

Interpreting chest x-rays of infants and children can be challenging. Normal anatomical structures in adults may look completely different in children and not be abnormal. Anatomical structures change with growth as children become older. Obtaining an adequate film on infants and children may also be challenging due to lack of cooperation or inability to follow commands.

In infants and small children, the heart may appear larger in size and take up the majority of the chest cavity. It may be difficult to visualize the pulmonary vasculature and pleura due to the size of the heart (Figure 4.20). The thymus may cause confusion and be mistaken for a mass in the upper chest in pediatric chest radiographs because it is readily visualized in infants and small children. However, as a child grows in size, the thymus remains the same size and eventually becomes obscured and not visible

(A)

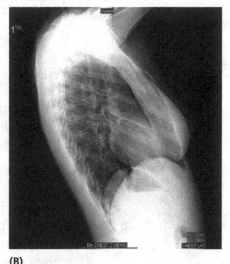

(B)

FIGURE 4.20 Comparing the child and adult chest x-rays: normal adult chest x-ray (A) and normal adult chest x-ray lateral (B).

(continued)

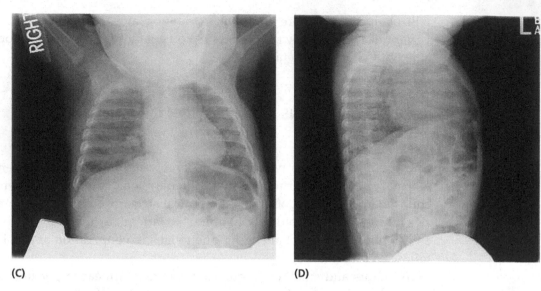

(C) (D)

FIGURE 4.20 *(continued)* Normal child chest x-ray (C) and normal child chest x-ray lateral (D).
Courtesy of Dr. David Begleiter.

in adult patient images. When viewing the skeleton of pediatric patients, the bones may not be as bright or white as in adults because they are more fibrous and not as calcified as mature bone with higher levels of calcium. Children also have growth plates at the epiphyseal regions of bones that may appear as fractures or breaks in the bony cortex, but these are normal ossification centers and will be discussed in detail in the extremity chapters.

MEDIASTINAL WIDTH

The mediastinum is the central thorax between the lungs and the heart and is divided into three regions: the anterior, middle, and posterior regions.

Anterior—area behind the sternum and in front of the heart and great vessels

Middle—area between the anterior and posterior pericardium that includes the pericardium, heart, aortic arch, proximal brachialcephalic vessels, pulmonary veins and arteries, trachea and main bronchi, and lymph nodes

Posterior—area behind the heart and trachea that includes the vertebral bodies

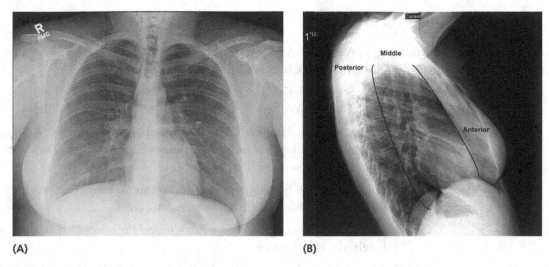

(A)

(B)

FIGURE 4.21 Normal mediastinal width (A) and widened mediastinum (B).
Courtesy of Dr. David Begleiter; diagramming, Theresa M. Campo.

Some literature includes the superior region that is above the heart and great vessels.

The aorta should be small and tight and not tortuous or widened (Figure 4.21). If the aorta is wide in appearance, the first thing that must be done is to make sure the film is adequate and you are looking at the proper view. If everything is acceptable, then consideration for a CT scan should be the next step to further evaluate the aorta and mediastinum for abnormalities.

CONCLUSION

The intention of this chapter was to introduce the reader to an approach to examining chest films. Chest radiograph interpretation can be intimidating, but once you are used to the geography of the chest, identification of normal and abnormal findings fall into place. Take each image one at a time, collaborate with colleagues and radiologists, and look at as many images as you can. One recommendation I give students is to look at the study and then read the radiologist's interpretation and compare. If the radiologist comments on something, look for it, so you will be familiar with that finding the next time you see it.

RESOURCES

Au-Yong, I., Au-Yong, A., & Broderick, N. (2010). *On-call x-rays made easy.* Philadelphia, PA: Churchill Livingstone, Elsevier.

Collins, J., & Stern, E. J. (2008). *Chest radiology: The essentials* (2nd ed.). Philadelphia, PA: Wolters Kluwer/Lippincott Williams & Wilkins.

Gay, S. B., Olazagasti, J., Higginbotham, J. W., Gupta, A., Wurm, A., & Nguyen, J. (n.d.). Introduction to chest radiology. Retrieved from https://www.med-ed .virginia.edu/courses/rad/cxr/Index.html

Goodman, L. R. (2015). *Felson's principles of chest roentgenology: A programmed text* (4th ed.). Philadelphia, PA: Elsevier Saunders.

Herring, W. (2016). *Learning radiology: Recognizing the basics* (3rd ed., pp. 8–34). Philadelphia, PA: Elsevier.

John, S. D., & Swischuk, L. E. (2012). Pediatric chest. In W. E. Brant & C. A. Helms (Eds.), *Fundamentals of diagnostic radiology* (4th ed., pp. 1128–1175). Philadelphia, PA: Wolters Kluwer/Lippincott Williams & Wilkins.

Klein, J. S. (2012). Mediastinum and hila. In W. E. Brant & C. A. Helms (Eds.), *Fundamentals of diagnostic radiology* (4th ed., pp. 367–396). Philadelphia, PA: Wolters Kluwer/Lippincott Williams & Wilkins.

Lemo, J., & Klein, J. S. (2012). Methods of examination, normal anatomy, and radiographic findings of chest disease. In W. E. Brant & C. A. Helms (Eds.), *Fundamentals of diagnostic radiology* (4th ed., pp. 324–366). Philadelphia, PA: Wolters Kluwer/Lippincott.

Mueller, J. S., & Daffner, R. H. (2014). Cardiac imaging. In R. H. Daffner & M. S. Hartman (Eds.), *Clinical radiology: The essentials* (4th ed., pp. 163–202). Philadelphia, PA: Wolters Kluwer/Lippincott Williams & Wilkins.

Mueller, J. S., & Daffner, R. H. (2014). Chest imaging. In R. H. Daffner & M. S. Hartman (Eds.), *Clinical radiology: The essentials* (4th ed., pp. 79–162). Philadelphia, PA: Wolters Kluwer/Lippincott Williams & Wilkins.

Shelton, D. K. (2012). Cardiac anatomy, physiology, and imaging modalities. In W. E. Brant & C. A. Helms (Eds.), *Fundamentals of diagnostic radiology* (4th ed., pp. 568–594). Philadelphia, PA: Wolters Kluwer/Lippincott Williams & Wilkins.

Abnormalities Found on Radiographs of the Chest

There are many abnormalities that can be identified on a chest radiograph. The intent of this chapter is to introduce some of the more common findings seen on a chest radiograph including atelectasis, pulmonary edema, pleural effusion, consolidation, pneumothorax, pneumomediastinum, hyperaeration, and masses. The more radiographs you review and evaluate, the more findings of normal variants and abnormalities you will be able to identify.

ATELECTASIS

Atelectasis is a condition of volume loss in a portion of the lung involving a subsegment, segment, lobe, or the entire lung. Atelectasis appears as a density or lighter area on the x-ray that is usually linear but may also have a curvilinear or wedge-shaped appearance on film. Atelectasis most commonly occurs from obstruction, usually of the bronchus by a mucous plug, neoplasm, or a foreign body. It may also be compressive and caused by a tumor, heart enlargement, hypoinflation, or emphysematous bullae. Patients who have had granulomatous disease such as tuberculosis, pulmonary infarct, or trauma may have scar tissue that can also cause atelectasis. It can be adhesive from the inactivation of surfactant or passive with the normal compliance of the lung within the pneumothorax or pleural effusion when the airway remains patent. Atelectasis may be present in one lobe or in multiple lobes. Because of the volume loss of air in the particular affected area, the findings on radiographs will be brighter/lighter shades of gray within the birdcage (see Figure 5.1).

FIGURE 5.1 Atelectasis.
Courtesy of Theresa M. Campo.

PULMONARY EDEMA

There are two basic types of pulmonary edema: cardiogenic and noncardiogenic. Cardiogenic pulmonary edema is caused by increased hydrostatic pulmonary capillary pressure, whereas noncardiogenic pulmonary edema is caused by an alteration in capillary membrane permeability or decreased plasma oncotic pressure. So just think of this simplistically: Cardiogenic is failure of the pump, whereas noncardiogenic is a problem with the plumbing leading to or from the heart.

Pulmonary edema may result in a variety of patterns on a plain radiograph of the chest. These include cephalization of the pulmonary vessels, Kerly A lines, Kerly B lines, peribronchial cuffing, bat wing pattern, patchy shadowing with an air bronchogram, heart enlargement, and/or pleural effusions (Figure 5.2).

(A)   **(B)**

FIGURE 5.2 Pulmonary edema (A) and pulmonary edema with pleural effusion cardiomegaly with mediastinum widening (B).
Copyright 2016. Dr. Frank Gaillard. Courtesy of Dr. Frank Gaillard and Radiopaedia.org. Used under license.

PLEURAL EFFUSION

Pleural effusions may be caused by congestive heart failure, infection, trauma, pulmonary embolus, tumor, autoimmune disease, ascites, and/or renal failure. Regardless of the cause, it is important to identify a pleural effusion and make the decision, based on clinical and diagnostic findings, whether the effusion needs to be treated. Pleural effusions can be identified using plain radiographs, but they may also be identified and further evaluated with CT scan and ultrasonography.

On an upright posterior–anterior (PA) image, blunting of the costophrenic angle(s) will be seen with a pleural effusion as fluid settles in the lowest or most dependent regions, which are the costophrenic angles. If a lateral decubitus image is obtained, identification of a pleural effusion can be made similarly by looking at a tabletop appearance to the affected lung. Large effusions can cause the mediastinum to shift away from the side of the effusion (Figure 5.3).

(A)   **(B)**

FIGURE 5.3 (A) and (B) demonstrate pleural effusion. Note the loss of the lower right birdcage especially the costophrenic angle.
Courtesy of Dr. David Begleiter.

INTERPRETATION OF INFILTRATES AND CONSOLIDATION

Infiltrates and consolidations are representative of opacities that are seen as bright or lighter gray to white on an image. What is important to know is the location of the opacity in identifying where the abnormality is. When we discussed the ABCs (*a*dequacy/*a*irway, *b*reathing or *b*irdcages, *c*ardiac/*c*irculation) of interpretation of the chest film, we evaluated the edges within our birdcages. The right heart border is adjacent to the right middle lobe and the right diaphragm is representative of the right lower lobe. The left heart border is adjacent to the left upper lobe and the left diaphragm to the left lower lobe (Figure 5.4). If these edges are not crisp and clear but are hazy or not identifiable, then you are visualizing an infiltrate or consolidation, which may represent a pneumonia, pneumonitis, or mass (see Figure 5.5). If an opacity is identified and clinically correlated, a diagnosis of pneumonia or pneumonitis is given. The patient then must have repeat films in 3 to 4 weeks demonstrating resolution. If there is little to no change or an increase in the identified opacity, then a CT scan may be ordered to further investigate the identified area, which may be representative of a mass or tumor.

When evaluating consolidation, one wants to note if the heart borders or diaphragm are obliterated or are shadowed by the area of consolidation. If the consolidation is located posterior to the heart, then the edges will not be obliterated. However, if the area of consolidation is anterior, it will obliterate the borders.

FIGURE 5.4 Chest x-ray with lobe borders.
Courtesy of Dr. David Begleiter; diagramming, Theresa M. Campo.

FIGURE 5.5 Infiltrates and consolidation right middle lobe and right lower lobe (A); right middle lobe and right lower lobe lateral view (B); normal triangle behind heart silhouette (C); left lower lobe (D); right middle lobe (E); right middle lobe lateral view (F).

(continued)

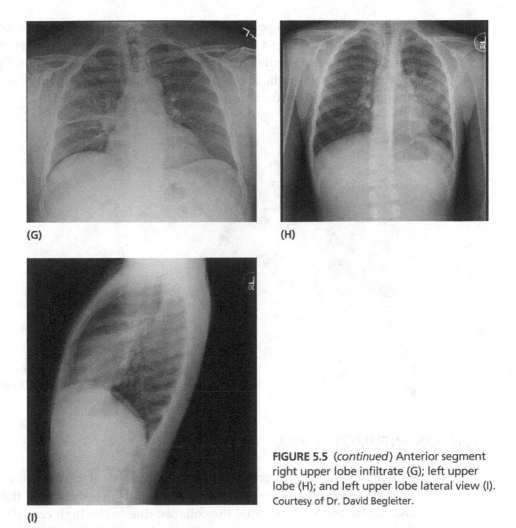

(G)

(H)

(I)

FIGURE 5.5 (*continued*) Anterior segment right upper lobe infiltrate (G); left upper lobe (H); and left upper lobe lateral view (I). Courtesy of Dr. David Begleiter.

PNEUMOTHORAX

Pneumothorax occurs when air inside the thoracic cavity becomes trapped outside the lung. Since the lung is a negative pressure system, any interruption within or outside of the system can cause a pneumothorax to occur. The mechanism of a pneumothorax results when inspired air escapes to an area outside the lung but within the chest cavity. This trapped air increases with each inspiration, resulting in increased intrathoracic pressure within the affected side; thus causing the lung to collapse.

A pneumothorax may be spontaneous, caused by blunt or penetrating trauma, or occur secondary to an invasive procedure such as surgery or central line placement. A pneumothorax can also be caused secondary to asthma or chronic obstructive pulmonary disease (COPD), bleb rupture, pulmonary infections, neoplasm, Marfan syndrome, or smoking cocaine. Findings on a radiograph indicative of a pneumothorax are absence of lung markings throughout the birdcage (Figure 5.6). This may be more apparent in the apices of the lung or top of the birdcage. A small pneumothorax may be identified by noting a darker shade of gray or black in the apex of one lung, which is representative of the air that is being trapped and pushing or replacing that particular segment of lung tissue. Identification of a pneumothorax is best demonstrated on an expiration view.

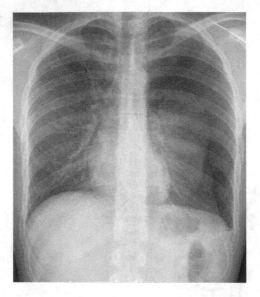

FIGURE 5.6 Pneumothorax.
Source: Hellerhoff (2010). https://commons.wikimedia.org/wiki/File:05-Spontanpneumothorax.jpg

TENSION PNEUMOTHORAX

If a pneumothorax extends or is left untreated, it can cause a tension pneumothorax. A tension pneumothorax results in a shifting of the trachea and mediastinum away from the collapse due to the high cavity pressure. This can be identified on a plain radiograph easily (Figure 5.7).

FIGURE 5.7 Tension pneumothorax.
Drawing by Jody Glenn.

PNEUMOMEDIASTINUM

Pneumomediastinum is free air that can be found within the mediastinum as well as the soft tissue of the chest cavity, chest wall, or neck (Figure 5.8). It can result from asthma, surgery, a traumatic tracheobronchial rupture, increased intrathoracic pressure, ruptured esophagus, barotrauma, or by smoking crack cocaine. On plain radiographs, streaky lucencies over the mediastinum may extend up into the neck or cause elevation of the parietal pleura along the mediastinal borders. It is important when looking at a chest x-ray to evaluate the entire image of the pleural cavity, including the neck and soft tissues, to identify possible free air.

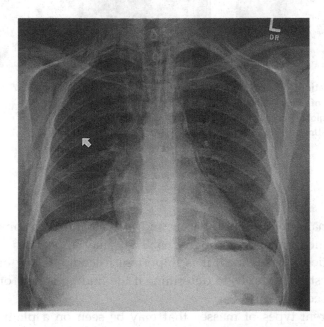

FIGURE 5.8 Pneumomediastinum. Reprinted by permission of James Heilman, MD, Wikipedian, ER Department Head, East Kootenay Regional Hospital, Clinical Assistant Professor, Department of Emergency Medicine, University of British Columbia.

HYPERAERATION

Hyperaeration may be caused by asthma or COPD producing both subtle and overt findings on plain radiographs. Emphysema causes a loss of normal elastic recoil of the lung and destruction of the pulmonary capillary bed and alveolar septa. Diffuse hyperinflation of the lungs can cause flattening of both diaphragms, increasing the retrosternal space. Radiographic findings include prominent central pulmonary artery vasculature with rapid tapering from decreased markings, giving a pruned appearance, hyperlucency due to increased aeration and lung volume, depression or "flattening" of the diaphragmatic curves, and blunting of the costophrenic angles (Figure 5.9).

FIGURE 5.9 Hyperaeration.
Reprinted by permission of James Heilman, MD, Wikipedian, ER Department
Head, East Kootenay Regional Hospital, Clinical Assistant Professor, Department
of Emergency Medicine, University of British Columbia.

MASSES AND TUMORS

Masses, or pulmonary nodules, of the lung and mediastinum are common
and can be identified on plain radiographs. They may appear as single
or multiple densities. If visualized, it is important to compare the image
with any prior chest radiographs to determine if the finding is new or has
changed or increased over time.

There are different types of masses that may be seen on a plain film
including cancer, abscesses, hematomas, cysts, lymphadenopathy, and
changes suggestive of lymphoma or tuberculosis. The diagnostic impres-
sion requires a thorough history and physical examination and may require
further testing to definitively identify the mass and its etiology.

It may be difficult to identify the exact location of a mass because the
mediastinum is arbitrarily divided into areas of overlapping structures and
compartments. Generally, masses in the mediastinum appear more clearly
than masses that originate in the lung and often compress or displace other
structures within the mediastinum. Masses originating in the lungs are usually surrounded by lung tissue and are less distinct. Once a mass is suspected, further diagnostic testing with CT scan or MRI may be needed to
confirm the exact type of lesion. Understanding how to differentiate types
of masses is beyond the intent of this text.

CONCLUSION

The ability to identify normal and abnormal findings on a chest radiograph will become easier once you begin looking at them yourself. Comparing one's interpretation with a radiologist's final reading is an excellent way to improve your skills. If there is something identified or not identified by the radiologist, examine the films again. You may be able to visualize the area noted in the report, which will help you identify subtle findings on other images. Establishing a working relationship with radiology colleagues will also enhance your knowledge and proficiency.

RESOURCES

Au-Yong, I., Au-Yong, A., & Broderick, N. (2010). *On-call x-rays made easy*. Philadelphia, PA: Churchill Livingstone, Elsevier.

Collins, J., & Stern, E. J. (2008). *Chest radiology: The essentials* (2nd ed.). Philadelphia, PA: Wolters Kluwer/Lippincott Williams & Wilkins.

Goodman, L. R. (2015). *Felson's principles of chest roentgenology: A programmed text* (4th ed.). Philadelphia, PA: Elsevier Saunders.

Green, C. E., & Klein, J. S. (2012). Pulmonary vascular disease. In W. E. Brant & C. A. Helms (Eds.), *Fundamentals of diagnostic radiology* (4th ed., pp. 396–409). Philadelphia, PA: Wolters Kluwer/Lippincott Williams & Wilkins.

Herring, W. (2016). *Learning radiology: Recognizing the basics* (3rd ed., pp. 35–84, 97–113). Philadelphia, PA: Elsevier.

Klein, J. S. (2012). Airway disease. In W. E. Brant & C. A. Helms (Eds.), *Fundamentals of diagnostic radiology* (4th ed., pp. 487–503). Philadelphia, PA: Wolters Kluwer/Lippincott Williams & Wilkins.

Klein, J. S. (2012). Pulmonary infection. In W. E. Brant & C. A. Helms (Eds.), *Fundamentals of diagnostic radiology* (4th ed., pp. 435–452). Philadelphia, PA: Wolters Kluwer/Lippincott Williams & Wilkins.

Klein, J. S. (2012). Pulmonary neoplasm. In W. E. Brant & C. A. Helms (Eds.), *Fundamentals of diagnostic radiology* (4th ed., pp. 410–434). Philadelphia, PA: Wolters Kluwer/Lippincott Williams & Wilkins.

Klein, J. S., & Ghostine, J. S. (2012). Pulmonary vascular disease. In W. E. Brant & C. A. Helms (Eds.), *Fundamentals of diagnostic radiology* (4th ed., pp. 504–535). Philadelphia, PA: Wolters Kluwer/Lippincott Williams & Wilkins.

Klein, J. S., & Green, C. E. (2012). Diffuse lung disease. In W. E. Brant & C. A. Helms (Eds.), *Fundamentals of diagnostic radiology* (4th ed., pp. 453–486). Philadelphia, PA: Wolters Kluwer/Lippincott Williams & Wilkins.

Mueller, J. S., & Daffner, R. H. (2014). Chest imaging. In R. H. Daffner & M. S. Hartman (Eds.), *Clinical radiology: The essentials* (4th ed., pp. 79–162). Philadelphia, PA: Wolters Kluwer/Lippincott Williams & Wilkins.

6

Basic Interpretation of the Abdomen

Abdominal radiographs can be beneficial in evaluating for intestinal perforation and small and large bowel obstruction, as well as for identifying foreign bodies and renal calculi. Traditionally, radiographs were used in diagnosing these disorders; however, with the advent and progression of technology, other studies may be utilized such as ultrasound, CT scan, or MRI. The benefit to abdominal radiographs is they are inexpensive and easily obtained.

An adequate, well-penetrated, erect abdominal x-ray, as well as the use of the left decubitus view (if the patient is unable to sit or stand), can identify as little as 1 mL of free air. To evaluate an obstruction, the erect chest x-ray and supine abdominal view are not only beneficial in identifying an obstruction but also reveal infiltrates or consolidation in the lower lobes of the lungs, which may be the source of abdominal pain. The supine view is also beneficial in identifying renal calculi. However, some facilities are replacing the use of plain films with CT scan without contrast to not only rule out stones but also evaluate for hydronephrosis.

Consideration of cost for patients who are underinsured or have no insurance may lead to utilizing plain radiographs to evaluate if stones are present. An obstruction series can be beneficial in identifying radiopaque foreign bodies that are either ingested or placed in the anus or vagina. It can also be used to track the progression, or lack thereof, of an already established ureteral stone. CT has become exclusively used in many facilities; plain radiographs are not only important, but they are cost effective. It is important to have a firm foundation and knowledge of anatomy, physiology, and pathophysiology when reviewing any radiographic study.

INTERPRETATION AND NORMAL FINDINGS

To begin the interpretation of abdominal films, one must utilize the ABCs. The ABCs for abdominal films are slightly different from those used when evaluating chest films. The ABCs allow you to identify normal from abnormal with an organized consistent approach. The ABCs are:

*A*dequacy/*A*ir—free intraperitoneal air rises to the anterior region of the abdomen (front of the abdomen) when the patient is supine, so it is best viewed on erect films if a perforation is suspected (Figure 6.1). Remember, hot air rises and can identify the presence of intraperitoneal air as well as intestinal air–fluid levels (Figure 6.2). Visualize the small and large intestines and assess air–fluid levels and caliber of the intestinal lumen.

FIGURE 6.1 Intraperitoneal air.
Courtesy of Dr. Douglas W. Parrillo.

FIGURE 6.2 Intestinal air–fluid levels.
Courtesy of Dr. David Begleiter.

*B*owel gas patterns—the small bowel lies in the center of the abdomen. It is of smaller caliber, approximately 3 cm, than the colon and contains air and fluid. The large bowel lies peripherally and contains feces, especially in the distal aspects, and there is no definite measurement as it varies based on the stool content; however, it should not measure more than 5.5 cm. Haustra are present in the large bowel but not in small bowel, making it easy to differentiate the two. Gas and air rise anteriorly while in the supine position and are best viewed in the erect view, demonstrating air in the stomach, transverse colon, and sigmoid colon (Figure 6.3).

FIGURE 6.3 (A) through (D) demonstrate various bowel gas patterns.
Courtesy of Dr. David Begleiter.

Calcification—calcifications can be seen and may be normal or abnormal. Phleboliths, which are small calcified veins in the pelvis, are often confused with stones in the urinary tract. More than 90% of renal stones can be visualized on a plain film. In 10% to 15% of patients with gallstones, these stones can also be visualized on a plain film (Figure 6.4).

FIGURE 6.4 Calcifications/stones. Note the various densities above the pelvis and within the main ring of the pelvis.
Courtesy of Bill Rhodes/Wikipedia Commons.

*D*ensities—radiopaque foreign bodies, whether ingested or inserted, can be identified on plain radiographs as radiographic densities (Figure 6.5).

FIGURE 6.5 Foreign body.
Source: Pandey, Dang, and Healy (2005).

*E*dges—The bowel and gastric folds can be identified and aid in identifying abnormal findings. The bowel wall should not be more than 3 mm thick. The small and large bowel should not be more than 3 cm in diameter and the cecum should never exceed 9 cm in diameter. Gastric folds should be parallel to the long axis of the stomach and the small bowel folds should be followed from one side to the other. In the large bowel, the haustral folds do not go from side to side but go partially across on each side; however, they do not meet (Figure 6.6).

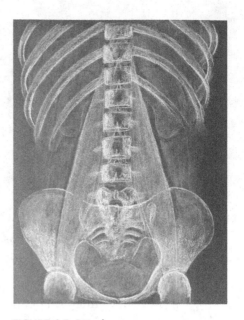

FIGURE 6.6 Edges (A is the kidney; B, the lung; C, the psoas muscle; and D, the bladder).
Drawing by Jodi Glenn.

FIGURE 6.7 Fat planes.
Drawing by Jodi Glenn.

*F*at plane—fat plane may be normally visualized on the abdominal radiographs but often represent an abnormality. If a fat plane is identified in the psoas, perirenal, perivesical, or retroperitoneal areas, this is considered to be abnormal and must be further evaluated with other diagnostic studies (Figure 6.7).

*S*keleton, solid organs—it is important to evaluate the skeleton throughout the abdominal series to identify any occult or obvious fractures (Figure 6.8). Depending on the location and extent of the fracture, underlying organ damage must be considered. If fractures of varying age are identified, abuse must be given consideration.

FIGURE 6.8 Skeletal fracture on abdominal film.
Source: Theresa M. Campo.

FREE AIR AND AIR–FLUID LEVELS

Intraluminal gas patterns and free air can be indicative of bowel obstruction or pneumoperitoneum. Intraluminal gas patterns can either be balanced and occur at the same level or at different levels (stair-step) (Figure 6.9). Abnormally produced intraluminal air–fluid levels in more than one bowel loop, distention, and the presence of mucosal wall thickening are indicative of an obstruction.

FIGURE 6.9 (A) through (D) demonstrate intraluminal gas patterns of obstruction. Note the air/fluid levels and paucity of markings distal to the obstruction.

Courtesy of Dr. Douglas W. Parrillo.

In the colon, air mixed with bowel contents can give a bubbly appearance and may be normal in adults, but is never normal in children and infants. Gaseous distention of the small or large bowel with air–fluid levels may be indicative of an ileus. When obstruction occurs, the bowel loops proximal to the obstruction, becomes distended/dilated, and there is paucity of gas distal to the obstruction. Distention can be significant. In the pediatric patient, intussusception can give a mass effect, target appearance (telescoping of bowel), and crescent streaking of air that outlines the trapped bowel (Figure 6.10).

(A)

(B)

(C)

FIGURE 6.10 (A) through (C) demonstrate intussusception.
Source: Images reprinted with permission from Medscape Drugs & Diseases (2016), available at http://emedicine.medscape.com/article/930708-overview

Extraluminal gas or free air can be indicative of a pneumoperitoneum and is best visualized on an erect film (Figure 6.11). If the patient is unable to sit or stand, then a lateral decubitus view can be obtained to identify the free air. Extraluminal air can be present in an abscess, retroperitoneal space, or bowel wall under the diaphragm or biliary or portal venous system of the liver. Perforation of viscous can be either intraperitoneal or retroperitoneal. The most common cause of pneumoperitoneum is either a perforated peptic ulcer or colonic diverticulum.

(A)

(B)

(C)

FIGURE 6.11 (A) through (C) demonstrate pneumoperitoneum.
Copyright 2016. Dr. Alexandra Stanislavsky.
Image courtesy of Dr. Alexandra Stanislavsky and Radiopaedia.org. Used under license.

CALCIFICATIONS

Calculi are readily visualized on abdominal films because the majority are made up of calcium or cholesterol, which can be easily visualized on radiographs. Calcifications, representing renal calculi, may be identified along the urinary tract from the kidneys down to the urethra. Gallstones can be seen within the gallbladder, and calcifications within vessels are known as fecoliths (Figure 6.4).

FOREIGN BODIES

Foreign bodies in the gastrointestinal tract and genitourinary tract may be ingested or inserted. Plain radiographs of the abdomen are beneficial only if the foreign body is radiopaque and has either a high-density or a metallic component within it. The object will appear as a bright white color on the film and, depending on its location, may look out of place when considering the mode in which it arrived in the area (Figure 6.5).

DILATED SMALL BOWEL

The most common cause of dilated small bowel is mechanical obstruction and paralytic ileus. Mechanical obstruction may be caused by adhesions, strangulated hernia, mass, gallstones, Crohn's disease-related strictures, appendiceal abscess, volvulus, or intussusception. When evaluating the abdominal plain radiograph, the normal caliber of the small intestine should not be greater than 3 cm. If the small bowel is dilated greater than 3 cm and contains variable air and fluid levels and the large bowel is not dilated or not able to be visualized, then an obstruction must be suspected. The small bowel will have the appearance of a "string of beads" when air gets trapped between the valvulae conniventes (Figure 6.12). If a small bowel obstruction is suspected, then a CT scan should be considered for further investigation into the cause and extent of the obstruction.

FIGURE 6.12 Small bowel obstruction. Reprinted by permission of James Heilman, MD, Wikipedian, ER Department Head, East Kootenay Regional Hospital, Clinical Assistant Professor, Department of Emergency Medicine, University of British Columbia.

DILATED LARGE BOWEL AND MEGACOLON

The large bowel may be visualized on the abdominal film. When large bowel dilatation is present, the colonic diameter is greater in caliber, measuring 5.5 cm, and is considered to be abnormal (Figure 6.13). Large bowel dilatation may occur with or without an obstruction and may be caused by tumors, volvulus, inflammatory bowel disease, diverticulitis, or other forms of colitis. Volvulus most often occurs in the cecum and sigmoid colon. Perforation of the colon must be considered in patients with volvulus when the caliber of the lumen exceeds 9 cm. When large bowel dilatation occurs in patients with inflammatory bowel disease, characterized by wall thickening with mucosal edema, toxic megacolon must be considered. Thumb printing can be seen on obstruction series, suggesting possible microscopic or overt perforation (Figure 6.14). If a large bowel obstruction is suspected, then a CT scan should be considered for further evaluation. Contrasted radiographs should not be considered or used with large bowel obstruction. The barium sulfate does not dilute and can worsen an obstruction and also obscure visualization with CT scan for further evaluation.

FIGURE 6.13 Large bowel dilation.
Reprinted by permission of James Heilman, MD, Wikipedian, ER Department Head, East Kootenay Regional Hospital, Clinical Assistant Professor, Department of Emergency Medicine, University of British Columbia.

FIGURE 6.14 Megacolon.
Source: Hellerhoff (2012). https://commons.wikimedia.org/wiki/File:Toxisches_Megacolon_bei_Colitis_ulcerosa.jpg

CONCLUSION

Plain abdominal radiographs can be beneficial in identifying numerous abnormalities such as free air and fluid, obstruction, perforation, foreign bodies, and calcifications within the abdominal cavity. Plain films of the abdomen are also beneficial because they are less expensive than other radiographic studies such as CT scans and MRIs. However, with the progression of technology, other more expensive testing modalities may be adopted as first-line approaches. If the patient is a woman of childbearing age or a pediatric patient, ultrasound may be a beneficial alternative to abdominal radiography.

RESOURCES

Au-Yong, I., Au-Yong, A., & Broderick, N. (2010). *On-call x-rays made easy.* Philadelphia, PA: Churchill Livingstone, Elsevier.

Brant, W. E. (2012). Abdomen and pelvis. In W. E. Brant & C. A. Helms (Eds.), *Fundamentals of diagnostic radiology* (4th ed., pp. 670–691). Philadelphia, PA: Wolters Kluwer/Lippincott Williams & Wilkins.

Brant, W. E. (2012). Liver, biliary tree and gallbladder. In W. E. Brant & C. A. Helms (Eds.), *Fundamentals of diagnostic radiology* (4th ed., pp. 692–719). Philadelphia, PA: Wolters Kluwer/Lippincott Williams & Wilkins.

Brant, W. E. (2012). Mesenteric small bowel. In. W. E. Brant & C. A. Helms (Eds.), *Fundamentals of diagnostic radiology* (4th ed., pp. 765–779). Philadelphia, PA: Wolters Kluwer/Lippincott Williams & Wilkins.

Brant, W. E. (2012). Stomach and duodenum. In W. E. Brant & C. A. Helms (Eds.), *Fundamentals of diagnostic radiology* (4th ed., pp. 752–764). Philadelphia, PA: Wolters Kluwer/Lippincott Williams & Wilkins.

Brant, W. E., & Erickson, S. (2012). Colon and appendix. In W. E. Brant & C. A. Helms (Eds.), *Fundamentals of diagnostic radiology* (4th ed., pp. 780–795). Philadelphia, PA: Wolters Kluwer/Lippincott Williams & Wilkins.

Gay, S. B., Lambert, D. L., & Reynolds, R. (n.d.). Introduction to abdominal plain radiographs. Retrieved from https://www.med-ed.virginia.edu/courses/rad/PlainAbdomen/index.html

Hartman, M. S., & Daffner, R. H. (2014). Abdominal radiographs. In R. H. Daffner & M. S. Hartman (Eds.), *Clinical radiology: The essentials* (4th ed., pp. 215–251). Philadelphia, PA: Wolters Kluwer/Lippincott Williams & Wilkins.

Herring, W. (2016). *Learning radiology: Recognizing the basics* (3rd ed., pp. 129–139, 183–192). Philadelphia, PA: Elsevier.

Moshiri, S., & Brant, W. E. (2012). Pharynx and esophagus. In W. E. Brant & C. A. Helms (Eds.), *Fundamentals of diagnostic radiology* (4th ed., pp. 734–751). Philadelphia, PA: Wolters Kluwer/Lippincott Williams & Wilkins.

Pandey, B. B., Dang, T. C., & Healy, J. F. (2005). Embolic stroke complicating *Staphylococcus aureus* endocarditis circumstantially linked to rectal trauma from foreign body: A first case report. *BMC Infectious Diseases, 5*, 42. doi:10.1186/1471-2334-5-42. Retrieved from https://commons.wikimedia.org/wiki/File:Rectal_foreign_body_04.jpg

Interpretation of Extremity Radiographs

Basic Interpretation of Long Bone—Upper Extremity Radiographs

Radiographs of long bones, whether of the upper extremity or the lower extremity, are usually performed after a traumatic injury. However, pain, swelling, and/or redness may also be an indication for obtaining radiographs to rule out an abnormal growth, bursitis, and foreign bodies. Plain radiographs of long bones are beneficial in identifying fractures, subluxation, dislocation, and soft tissue swelling in traumatic injuries and are also useful in evaluating nontraumatic signs and symptoms such as abnormal bone growths.

In this chapter, normal findings on plain radiographs are discussed along with joint structures and normal variants, as well as common findings in adults and children. Knowledge of normal anatomical structures is imperative in interpreting long-bone radiographs.

NORMAL

Before ordering a plain radiograph of a long bone or joint, it is important to review some of the rules discussed in earlier chapters. Additionally, when evaluating the upper extremity, it is important to not only evaluate the affected area, but also the joints above and below. For instance, if the patient complains of an injury to the forearm, medical imaging should include the elbow as well as the wrist. Routine studies should include a minimum of two views; most have three views or more, depending on the area in question.

Plain radiographs are excellent in identifying bony abnormalities such as fractures. Although not the best modality for evaluating soft tissue conditions surrounding a particular joint, such as cartilage, muscle, and tendons, which are best seen using MRI, plain films do show changes within joint alignment and edema, which are indicative of an occult bone fracture, trauma, or inflammation. An example of an occult fracture finding is when the posterior fat pad, which is only visible if bleeding occurs within the joint space, is viewed on the lateral view of an elbow and the anterior fat pad appears like the sail of a sailboat, which is suggestive of a radial head fracture that may not be seen in the bony cortex (Figure 7.1).

 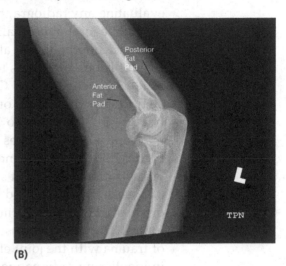

(A)   (B)

FIGURE 7.1 Anterior and posterior (A) and lateral (B) fat pad sign elbow.
Courtesy of Dr. Douglas W. Parrillo; diagramming, Theresa M. Campo.

The upper extremity consists of the shoulder, elbow, wrist, and phalangeal joints and associated bones: humerus, radius, ulna, carpal, metacarpal, and phalanges. Each joint and each bone have different appearances as well as functions within the upper extremity. Abnormalities can cause inhibition of normal function and use of the upper extremity. There are five types of bones in the body, as shown in Table 7.1. When evaluating bones on a radiograph, scan the cortical margins and note alignment to identify an abnormality.

TABLE 7.1 Five Types of Bones, Definition, and Examples

Type of Bone	Definition	Example
Long bone	The length is greater than the width	Femur, humerus, phalanges
Short bone	The length and width are comparable	Cuboid bones, carpals, tarsals

(continued)

TABLE 7.1 Five Types of Bones, Definition, and Examples (*continued*)

Type of Bone	Definition	Example
Flat bone	Diploic bones	Skull
Sesmoid bone	Small round bones that are located in tendons	Foot and hand
Irregular bone	Irregularly shaped	Vertebrae, sacrum

The ABCs of interpretation can be utilized for systematic assessment of the upper extremity. *A* is for *a*dequacy and *a*lignment. As stated in previous chapters, adequacy of the film is of the utmost importance when evaluating any radiographs. Proper alignment allows the viewer to identify subtle joint abnormalities. It does not only refer to the alignment of one particular bone, but also alignment within the joint (see Figure 7.2A). *B* is for *b*ones and refers to the evaluation of all components of the bone in the respective study. Cortical margins and borders should be evaluated for any disruption or lack of continuity of that bone indicative of a fracture. It also refers to any abnormal growths or appearances, which may appear as densities or opacities on the radiographic image (see Figure 7.2B). *C*artilage and joints can be evaluated for abnormalities with visualization of the joint space. Loss of any joint space may be indicative of a crush injury or could be a sign of degenerative joint disease. Bulging or displacement of normal structures in the lower extremity may be indicative of a joint effusion (see Figure 7.2C). *S*oft tissue can give signs of trauma with the joint effusion or edema. It can also assist the provider in identifying radiopaque foreign bodies that may have occurred during the injury itself.

FIGURE 7.2 Alignment of upper extremity bones (A); intact bony cortex (B); and joint space (C). Drawing courtesy of Theresa M. Campo.

ABNORMALITIES OF THE UPPER EXTREMITY

Fractures

Describing Fractures

A fracture or break to a bone, or bones, can happen from injury or pathology. Simply describing a fracture is important when documenting findings, but it is also important to utilize the proper terminology when describing these findings. A fracture line or pattern may be transverse, oblique, spiral, comminuted, impacted, avulsed, compressed, or depressed. A fracture may only involve one side of the bone, may involve both sides, or may go completely through the bone itself (see Figure 7.3). A normal variant that may be visualized involves blood vessels along the bone appearing as fractures. These can be differentiated from a fracture by tracing the lines and seeing if they pass the normal border of the bone (cortex). However, it is important to note that both may go through the cortex; many vascular channels traverse the cortex and make differentiating difficult.

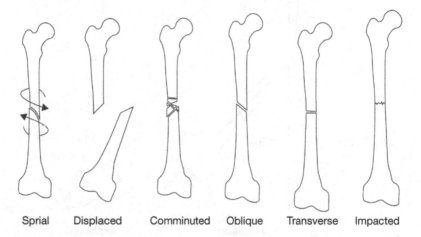

| Sprial | Displaced | Comminuted | Oblique | Transverse | Impacted |

FIGURE 7.3 Fracture patterns.
Drawing by Ocean City High School student.

Fractures may involve one bone or multiple bones. There may also be multiple fractures within the same bone but in different areas. The bone fragments may be displaced or nondisplaced. When a bone fragment is 100% displaced, causing shortening and overlapping of the bone fragments, this is known as a bayonet deformity (Figure 7.4). When the bone fragments are out of alignment of each other, they are considered to be angulated. Angulation is the angle between the longitudinal axis of the main fracture fragment and the other fragment. Significant angulation requires reduction and realignment of the bone fragments. If the fracture line is forced into the joint space, it is considered to be an intra-articular fracture (Figure 7.5).

A stress fracture can occur with repetitious loading beyond the bone tolerance. An avulsion fracture may occur when there is a forcible muscular

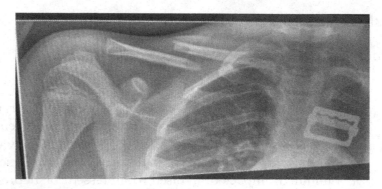

FIGURE 7.4 Bayonet deformity.
Courtesy of Theresa M. Campo.

Angulation   Displaced   Bayonet

FIGURE 7.5 Angulation, displacement, and a bayonet deformity.
Drawing by Ocean City High School student.

contraction of tendinous (tendon attaches muscle to bone, whereas ligament attaches bone to bone) attachment to a bone that is pulled off and away from the main structure.

Pediatric Considerations

Special consideration needs to be given with the pediatric patient. Pediatric bones are more fibrous and less crystalline (or calcified) than adult bones. They are enclosed in a sheet of strong fibrous periosteum and have epiphyseal growth plates, which are a zone of weakness. Children tend to have incomplete fractures such as a greenstick fracture or torus fracture because the bone ends do not separate as in adults because of the strong periosteal sleeve. The most common types of fractures in the pediatric patient are elastic deformation, bowing deformation, torus or buckle fracture, greenstick fracture, Salter–Harris fracture, stress injury, and avulsion injury (Figure 7.6).

Pediatric bones have epiphyseal growth plates that allow the bones to grow until they are mature adult bones. When a fracture occurs within or around the growth plate, it can complicate the healing process. Gross disturbances can be expected and the potential for loss of growth of the long bones may occur. However, current literature demonstrates that the loss of length after a fracture of a long bone tends to be made up in 1 to 2 years after the injury by overgrowth. The epiphyseal growth plate is a zone of weakness that can make fracture, separation, and slipping of the growth plate more common in the pediatric patient.

The Salter–Harris classification system is used to describe the five different types of pediatric growth plate fractures based on abnormalities involving either the metaphysis, epiphysis, and/or diaphysis. A Salter I fracture is a separation of the growth plate without involvement of the metaphysis or the epiphysis. A Salter II fracture occurs across the growth plate but with a small fragment of metaphysis remaining attached to the epiphysis. A fracture

Normal   Torus   Greenstick

FIGURE 7.6 Pediatric fractures.
Drawing by Ocean City High School student.

across the growth plate with extension of the fracture line across the epiphysis is known as a Salter III fracture. When the fracture line traverses the epiphysis and part of the diaphysis, this is known as a Salter IV fracture. Finally, when there is damage to both the epiphysis and the metaphysis from a crush injury this is known as a Salter V fracture. As you will notice, the severity of the injury, increases with the designating number of the Salter–Harris fracture (see Figure 7.7). An easy mnemonic to remember the Salter classification is SALTR. *s* refers to a *slip* as in a Salter I, *a* refers to the fracture noted *above* or proximal to the epiphyseal plate, *l* refers to a fracture be*low* or distal to the epiphyseal plate, *t* is a fracture line extending *through* the epiphyseal plate including both the epiphysis and metaphysis, and *r* refers to *crush*.

FIGURE 7.7 Five types of Salter–Harris fractures.
Drawing by Ocean City High School student.

Shoulder

Alignment of the glenohumeral joint should demonstrate the humeral head lying in the glenoid fossa, and the distance between the humeral head in the anterior margin of the glenoid should be equal from top to bottom (Figure 7.8). If the humeral head is internally rotated and looks like a light bulb, on a plain radiograph, suspect a posterior dislocation. Alignment of the acromioclavicular joint should show alignment of the inferior margins of the lateral end of the clavicle and acromium.

The shoulder is made up of three bones: the clavicle, the humerus, and the scapula. The scapula provides support and stability to the shoulder through three structures where tendons and ligaments attach. The coracoid process is in the anterior plane of the shoulder blade and the acromion is in the posterior region. These structures are supported by the coracoacromial ligament. The humeral head is adjacent to the glenoid portion of the scapula and is supported by the muscles, tendons, and ligaments that make up the rotator cuff. This region is referred to as the glenohumeral joint. The distal aspect of the clavicle, adjacent to the acromium, comprises the acromiocla-vicular joint. A fracture of any of the bony structures within the shoulder or a soft tissue injury to the rotator cuff ligaments and/or tendons results in shoulder instability, loss of function, and pain (see Figure 7.8).

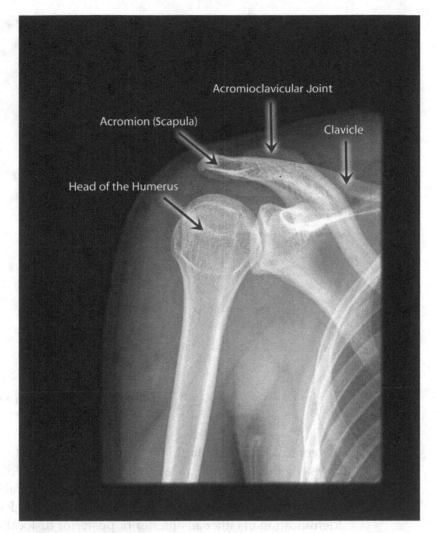

FIGURE 7.8 Shoulder anatomy.
Source: Campo and Lafferty (2016; Figure 42.1, p. 362).

Shoulder injuries are common in all age groups and may consist of a fracture, dislocation, or both occurring simultaneously. Clavicular fractures are the most common fractures in children and adolescents. Shoulder dislocation and acromioclavicular (AC) separations are most common in adults. In the elderly, the most common injury is fracture of the humerus, particularly the head and neck. If soft tissue injury is suspected and a dislocation and/or fracture has been ruled in or out with plain radiographs, an MRI should be considered for better visualization of the soft tissue structures.

Radiographic studies of the shoulder should have three views: the anterior–posterior (AP) view, axial view, and the "Y" view (Figure 7.9). The AP view allows for viewing the contour of each bone, which should be evaluated systematically. One should note that the cortices are smooth and visible ribs should also be evaluated. In the axial view, identification of

FIGURE 7.9 Three views of a shoulder radiograph.
Courtesy of Dr. David Begleiter.

the coracoid process should be visualized. The axial view is also useful in assessing the glenohumeral alignment for evaluation of any avulsions of the glenoid rim and for a Hill-Sachs defect of the humeral head. The "Y" view is beneficial for confirming normal alignment of the glenohumeral joint and identification of either an anterior or posterior dislocation.

As children grow and develop, so do their bones. There is formation of ossification centers of the humerus, scapula, and clavicle, which are formed over years and eventually fuse. Table 7.2 demonstrates the time of formation and time of fusion of the secondary ossification centers.

TABLE 7.2 Ossification Center Formation and Fusion

Shoulder Bone Ossification Center	Formation (years of age)	Fusion (years of age)
Humeral Head	< 6 months	16–18
Humerus - Greater Tuberosity	1	4–6
Humerus - Lesser Tuberosity	5	7
Scapula - Coracoid	1	20
Scapula - Inferior Angle	15	15
Scapula - Acromium	15	20–25
Clavicle - Medial Margin	18	25

Clavicle

Clavicle fractures can occur from minimal force and most often occur in the midshaft and distal aspect (Figure 7.10). Midshaft clavicle fractures may be seen more frequently in younger individuals, especially those younger than 20 or 21 years of age. Fractures of the lateral/distal aspects are more common in older individuals. The skin overlying a clavicle fracture should be assessed for tenting that is causing skin displacement. Tenting can result when fracture fragments protrude and pinch the skin. These fracture fragments may need to be repaired, requiring surgical intervention. One should suspect an intrathoracic injury with any proximal clavicle fracture, such as pneumothorax or pneumomediastinum.

(A)

(B)

(C)

FIGURE 7.10 Normal clavicle (A and B) and distal clavicle fracture (C).
Courtesy of Dr. David Begleiter.

Scapula

Fractures to the scapula incur a great deal of direct force and have a high correlation of injury to the thorax, head, and spine. When evaluating or identifying a scapular fracture, it is imperative that the provider completely evaluate all of the surrounding structures for accompanying injury. Scapular fractures can be difficult to identify and visualize on a plain radiograph. Obtaining a "Y" view is most beneficial, but MRI or CT scanning may be necessary for a definitive diagnosis (Figure 7.11).

(A)   (B)

FIGURE 7.11 Scapula fractures. Note in (A) and (B) the comminuted fracture with multiple bone fragments. (C) demonstrates the importance of more than one view for visualization of the fracture.
Courtesy of Dr. David Begleiter.

(C)

Humerus

There are four parts to the proximal humerus: the greater tuberosity, lesser tuberosity, head, and neck leading to the shaft (Figure 7.12). Proximal humeral fractures have a peak incidence during adolescence, causing epiphyseal separation. Fracture of this region in adults aged 45 years and older is most often due to osteoporosis. A fall with an outstretched hand is one of the more common mechanisms for fracture of the proximal humerus. If a fracture occurs in the humeral neck, it may be accompanied by complications from neurovascular injury, avascular necrosis, and adhesive capsulitis. A compression fracture of the posterolateral humeral head is known as a Hill–Sachs fracture and may be caused by anterior glenohumeral dislocation and impaction of the humeral head against the anterior glenoid rim.

Fractures to the shaft of the humerus may be complicated by injury to the radial nerve with entrapment or impingement. When a fracture occurs in the distal third of the humerus involving radial nerve entrapment, this is known as a Holstein–Lewis fracture (see Figure 7.13).

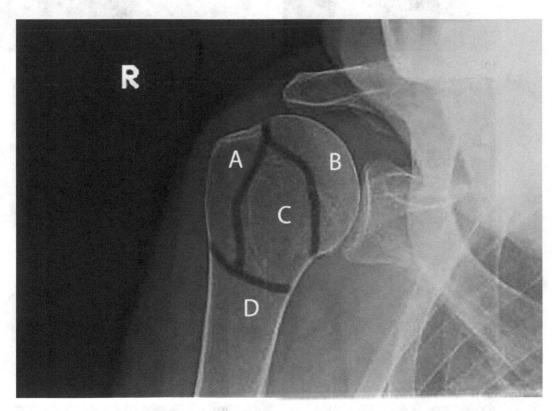

FIGURE 7.12 Four parts of the proximal humerus. Greater tuberosity (A); humeral head (B); lesser tuberosity (C); and humeral neck going into the shaft (D).
Courtesy of Dr. David Begleiter.

FIGURE 7.13 (A) through (D) demonstrate humerus fractures.
Courtesy of Dr. David Begleiter and Theresa M. Campo.

Elbow

The elbow joint consists of the distal humerus and the proximal radius and ulna. The distal humerus consists of the medial and lateral epicondyle, coronoid fossa, capitellum, and trochlea (Figure 7.14). The radial head, radial tuberosity, ulnar tuberosity, and olecranon process are key areas when evaluating an elbow image. The ulna and olecranon process articulate with the trochlea and the olecranon fossa of the humerus. The radial head articulates with the capitellum and the two structures should be aligned in all projections. Trauma to the elbow occurs in all ages but most commonly in children. Elbow fractures in children require emergent orthopedic consultation to avoid permanent deformity and loss of function. It is important to obtain an AP, lateral, and two oblique views when imaging the elbow.

FIGURE 7.14 Three views of a normal elbow study.
Courtesy of Dr. David Begleiter.

As with the shoulder, the pediatric patient has ossification centers in the elbow joint that appear and fuse at different ages. It is important to know the sequence of the appearance as well as fusion of these ossification centers in order to identify normal from abnormal findings. The order of appearance can be easily remembered with the mnemonic CRITOE, which represents *c*apitellum, *r*adius, *i*nternal or medial epicondyle, *t*rochlea, *o*lecranon, and *e*xternal or lateral epicondyle (Figure 7.15). The ages that these ossification centers appear are highly variable and differ between individuals; however, a general guide or rule of thumb is to remember the following:

C = 1 year
R = 3 years
I = 5 years
T = 7 years
O = 9 years
E = 11 years

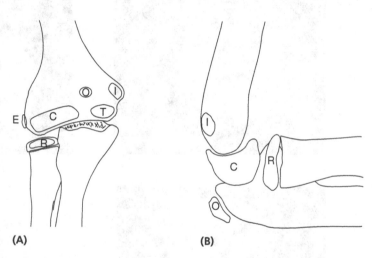

(A) (B)

FIGURE 7.15 Elbow ossification centers (CRITOE). Anterior–posterior view equivalent (A) and lateral view equivalent (B).
Drawings by Theresa M. Campo.

Evaluating alignment in the pediatric patient is also important because of the epiphyseal growth plates. The radiocapitellar line is a line drawn through the long axis of the radius that should always point toward the center of the capitellum regardless of the position of the patient since the radius articulates with the capitellum (Figure 7.16). When a dislocation occurs of the radius, the line will not pass through the center of the capitellum. An anterior humeral line is a line that can be drawn on a lateral view along the anterior surface of the humerus and should pass through the middle third of the capitellum (Figure 7.16). With a supracondylar fracture, the anterior humeral line will pass through the anterior third of the capitellum or directly in front of the capitellum due to posterior bending of the distal humeral fragment.

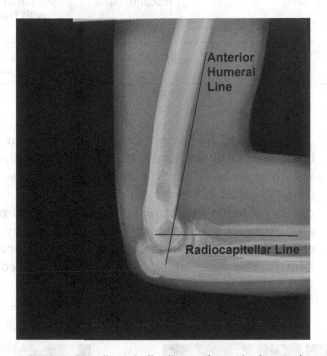

FIGURE 7.16 Radiocapitellar line and anterior humeral line and fracture. Note the anterior humeral line along the anterior aspect of the humerus through the capitellum and the radiocapitellar line traversing the capitellum and intersecting the proximal radius.
Courtesy of Dr. David Begleiter; diagramming,
Theresa M. Campo.

Fractures to the distal humerus can involve either the medial condyle or lateral condyle and can be very severe. Fracture of either one or both epicondyles can lead to long-term complications and disability of elbow movement. Fractures can occur anywhere within or above the condyles. Vascular and nerve injuries can occur with significantly displaced condylar fractures due to the brachial artery and median nerve, both lying anteriorly. Supracondylar fractures occurring in children are most commonly caused by a fall on outstretched hand (FOOSH) injury. Table 7.3 provides a description of various condylar fractures.

TABLE 7.3 Types of Condylar Fractures

Articular Location	Condyle	Fracture Location
Extra-articular	Epicondylar	Medial or lateral epicondyle
	Supracondylar	Above the epicondyle
Intra-articular	Transcondylar	Medial or lateral condyle fracture with fracture plane within the capsule
	Bicondylar	Fracture line splits the medial and lateral epicondyle

Radial head fractures most commonly occur from a FOOSH injury in adults. Occult fractures of the radial head may only be identified by visualization of fat pads. It can be normal to see a very small anterior fat pad located anterior to the coracoid. However, when the anterior fat pad is pushed outward and resembles the sail of a sailboat (known as a sail sign) and/or a posterior fat pad is easily visible, it is due to an effusion caused by leakage of blood from the bone and marrow into the joint. If these occur, an occult fracture must be considered and ruled out with further imaging (Figure 7.17).

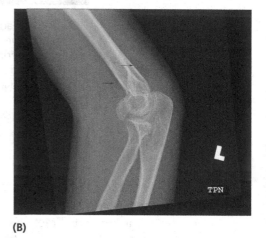

(A) **(B)**

FIGURE 7.17 (A), (B), (C), and (D) demonstrate a condylar fracture of the humerus with an anterior sail sign and posterior fat pad.
Courtesy of Dr. Douglas W. Parrillo; diagramming, Theresa M. Campo.

(continued)

(C)

(D)

FIGURE 7.17 (*continued*)
Courtesy of Dr. Douglas W. Parrillo.

Radius and Ulna

A distal radial fracture may occur solely or may be associated with dislocation of the distal radioulnar joint. This is commonly known as an Essex–Lopresti fracture (Figure 7.18). If the proximal third of the ulna is fractured with an associated dislocation of the radial head, this is known as a Monteggia fracture (Figure 7.19). The radius and ulna may be fractured anywhere along the shaft of one or both of these bones. Injury may result from either a direct blow to the posterior ulna or a fall with forceful pronation of the forearm. Radial head displacement into the antecubital fossa, elbow pain, and tenderness may be seen on clinical evaluation.

(A)

(B)

FIGURE 7.18 (A), (B), (C), and (D) demonstrate Essex–Lopresti fracture.

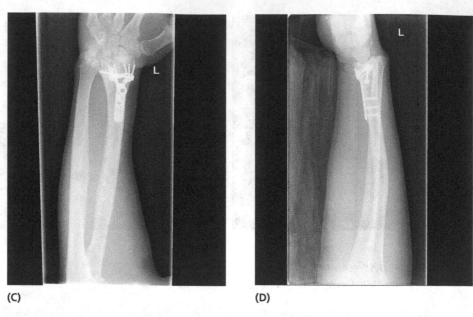

(C)   (D)

FIGURE 7.18 (*continued*)
Source: Courtesy of Dr. Henry Knipe Radiopaedia.org

FIGURE 7.19 Monteggia fracture.
Reprinted with permission from Medscape Drugs & Diseases (http://emedicine.medscape.com), 2016. Available at http://emedicine.medscape.com/article/1231438-overview

A Galeazzi fracture occurs when the proximal radius is fractured and associated with either subluxation or dislocation of the distal ulna (Figure 7.20). Barton's fracture occurs when there is displacement of the articular lip of the distal radius that may be associated with a carpal subluxation. A chauffeur's fracture, also known as a Hutchinson fracture, occurs when there is an intra-articular fracture of the radial styloid; this was named during the era of crank automobiles (Figure 7.21). A Colles fracture is when the fracture fragment of the distal radius is dorsally displaced with volar apex angulation (Figure 7.22). This fracture most often occurs from a FOOSH injury in elderly women. Approximately 50% of Colles fractures occur with an associated ulnar styloid fracture. When there is a distal radial fracture with volar displacement it is known as a Smith fracture.

FIGURE 7.20 Galeazzi fracture.
Courtesy of Hellerhoff/Wikipedia Commons.

(A)

(B)

FIGURE 7.21 (A) and (B) demonstrate chauffeur's fracture.
Copyright 2016. Dr. Alexandra Stanislavsky. Image courtesy of Dr. Alexandra Stanislavsky and Radiopaedia.org. Used under license.

(A)   **(B)**

FIGURE 7.22 (A) and (B) demonstrate a Colles fracture.
Courtesy of Dr. Douglas W. Parrillo.

Long-bone fractures in children that do not penetrate or break through the bony cortex are referred to as greenstick fractures. There are three types of greenstick fractures: transverse fractures occurring only half way through the bone; torus or buckle fractures where the cortex of the bone buckles and becomes overlapping; and bowing-bent bone when there is no identifiable bony cortex disruption but bowing of the bone is visualized (Figure 7.23).

Normal   Torus   Greenstick

FIGURE 7.23 Types of greenstick fractures.
Drawing by Ocean City High School student.

Carpals

Fractures may occur to any of the carpal bones; however, they are less frequently seen in comparison with metacarpal fractures and distal radius and ulna fractures. Carpal injuries are more commonly associated with separation and dislocation; in addition, fractures to the metacarpals and phalanges occur more frequently than fractures and dislocations of the carpal bones.

A triquetral fracture is the second most common carpal fracture, with scaphoid fracture being the most common. In this type of fracture, there is bone avulsion from the dorsal surface that is best viewed in the lateral view of the hand. Noting any soft tissue abnormalities of the dorsal wrist can also aid in identification of this fracture (Figure 7.24).

FIGURE 7.24 Triquetral fracture. Courtesy of Hellerhoff/Wikipedia Commons.

Scaphoid fractures, the most common carpal fractures, can be difficult to identify on radiographs (Figure 7.25). Obtaining a scaphoid view of the wrist may aid in identification along with assessing for tenderness in the anatomical snuff box region of the hand. This injury occurs with extreme dorsiflexion of the wrist and ulnar deviation. This type of fracture rarely occurs in children.

(A)

(B)

(C)

FIGURE 7.25 (A) through (C) demonstrate a scaphoid fracture.
Courtesy of Dr. Douglas W. Parrillo.

Metacarpals

One of the more common fractures of the hand is a boxer's fracture. This occurs during a punch-type injury or close-fisted impact, causing a fracture to the fifth metacarpal neck with volar displacement of the head of the metacarpal. Boxer's fractures may also involve the fourth metacarpal (Figure 7.26). These can become problematic injuries if there is open skin caused by a punch to another person's mouth with bacterial contamination from saliva. It is imperative that any punch injury with a bite and contamination from saliva or mucus be treated as an open fracture with antibiotic prophylaxis combined with close monitoring and orthopedic follow-up.

(A)

(B)

(C)

FIGURE 7.26 (A) through (C) demonstrate a Boxer's fracture.
Copyright 2016 Dr Henry Knipe. Image courtesy of Dr. Henry Knipe and
Radiopaedia.org. Used under license.

A Bennett's fracture is an intra-articular fracture—dislocation of the base of the first metacarpal. The separating triangular fragment most commonly dislocates dorsally (Figure 7.27). This type of fracture occurs from axial loading and most commonly occurs from a fight injury. Transverse or oblique are other common metacarpal fractures that may involve one or multiple metacarpals.

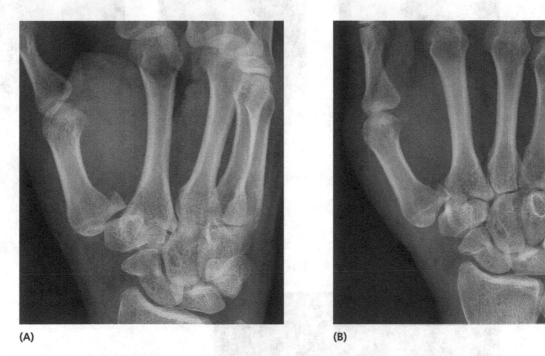

(A)   (B)

FIGURE 7.27 (A) and (B) demonstrate a Bennett's fracture.
Copyright 2016 Dr. Maulik S. Patel. Image courtesy of Dr. Maulik S. Patel and Radiopaedia.org. Used under license.

Phalanges

Fractures to the phalanges can be caused by crush injuries, jamming of the finger or fingers, or from direct trauma. Fractures to the distal phalanx need to be evaluated for possible nail plate and/or nail bed injury. Comminuted fractures of the tuft of the distal phalanx from a crushing injury may result in partial or full amputation of the distal finger (Figure 7.28).

Dislocations/Subluxations/Separations

Articular surfaces of bones within joints are kept in place by ligaments and cartilage. When the alignment of the adjacent bones is not maintained or they have lost complete contact with each other, then a subluxation or dislocation occurs. With a subluxation, the articular surface of one

(A)   (B)   (C)

(D)

FIGURE 7.28 Phalange fracture.
Fracture at the base of the fifth
proximal phalanx (A); fracture to the
middle phalanx (B and C); midshaft
fracture of fifth proximal phalnx (D).
Note the appliance to the third
proximal phalanx.
Courtesy of Kyle Deuter.

bone maintains contact with the articular surface of the adjacent bone. Although the bones are not in complete alignment, they have not lost contact with each other. When a dislocation occurs, the articular surface of one bone loses complete contact with the other, causing a complete disarticulation.

Shoulder

Dislocations occurring in the shoulder are most commonly either anterior, posterior, or inferior. For the purposes of this book, we will only discuss anterior and posterior dislocations, as inferior dislocations are less common. Anterior dislocations are most common, with posterior dislocation occurring in approximately 3% of all cases. Shoulder dislocations are the most commonly occurring due to the incredible range of motion and the anatomical structures that allow for such motion.

When evaluating any film, it is important to have an image in your mind of the normal anatomy. This is helpful when identifying dislocations of the shoulder. Visualize that the humeral head is sitting adjacent to the glenoid if the humeral head is shifted forward or anteriorly; it changes the appearance of the humeral head and proximal end of the humerus on radiograph. In the AP view, the head of the humerus will be under the coracoid and displaced toward the coracoid on the "Y" view. More than 95% of shoulder dislocation occurs anteriorly, with the displacement of the humeral head anterior to the glenoid cavity.

There are four types of anterior dislocations: subcoracoid, subglenoid, subclavicular, and intrathoracic, with the first two being the most commonly occurring. Anterior dislocations occur when indirect force to the arm is combined with abduction, extension, and external rotation of the arm. They may be accompanied by an impaction fracture of the anterior lip of the humeral head known as a Bankart fracture. Another commonly seen fracture associated with anterior dislocation is the Hill–Sachs defect, which is a fracture to the posterior–lateral aspect of the humeral head. This occurs when the humeral head is struck against the glenoid (Figure 7.29).

If the humeral head is shifted backward and is facing posteriorly, again, it changes the appearance of the humerus on a radiograph. With a posterior dislocation, the humeral head and proximal end of the humerus will have the appearance of a light bulb, especially in the AP view, and will be outside of the Y of the scapula on the "Y" view. There may be widening of the joint, usually greater than 6 mm, due to the lateral displacement of the humeral head. With approximately 3% of dislocations occurring posteriorly, they are very uncommon. It is caused by internal rotation and adduction from an indirect force. It may occur during a seizure, fall, or electrical/lightning shock. This type of dislocation may be difficult to identify on plain radiographs. Obtaining an axillary view is most beneficial (Figure 7.30).

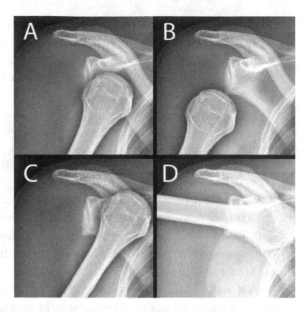

FIGURE 7.29 Four types of anterior dislocation: subcoracoid (A); subglenoioid (B); subclavicular (C); and intrathoracic (D).
Source: Campo and Lafferty (2016).

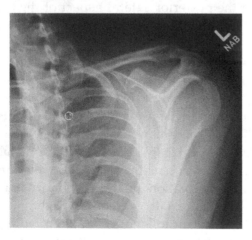

FIGURE 7.30 Three views demonstrating a posterior dislocation.
Source: Theresa M. Campo.

Injury to the acromioclavicular ligament can cause a separation between the acromium and the clavicle. There are three grades of separation and they are:

Grade I—Minimal displacement of the joint may be visualized on radiograph. There is stretching and possibly partial tearing of the acromioclavicular ligament. This is the most common type of injury to this joint.

Grade II—The acromioclavicular ligament is completely torn but the coracoclavicular ligaments remain intact. This may be apparent on the radiographs as a widening of the acromioclavicular space. However, it may not be obvious during a physical exam.

Grade III—Complete separation of the joint occurs when the acromioclavicular and coracoclavicular ligaments are torn and there is damage to the surrounding capsule. This will be an obvious finding on the radiograph with widening of the acromioclavicular space. Clinically, a bump on the shoulder may be palpated due to the clavicle being pushed upward while the weight of the arm causes the shoulder to fall (see Figure 7.31).

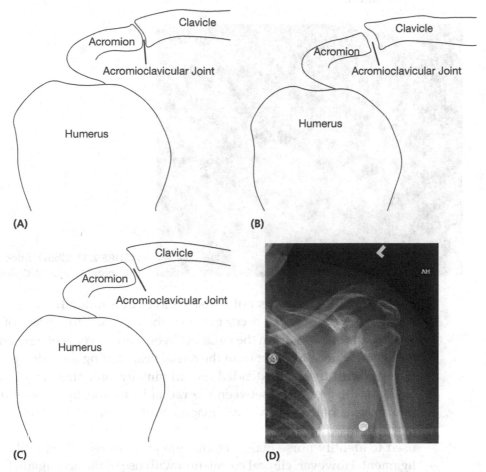

FIGURE 7.31 Three grades of acromioclavicular (AC) separation; grade I (A); grade II (B); and grade III (C). Grade III AC separation on radiograph (D).

Drawings courtesy of Theresa M. Campo. Image courtesy of Dr. Douglas W. Parrillo.

Elbow

The elbow is a large hinge joint that has two articulations. The first articulation is formed between the humerus and the ulna, which allows for flexion and extension. The second articulation is between the radius and humerus, which allows for supination and pronation. The elbow is stabilized by distinctive bony structures and ligaments that protect the joint from varying degrees of forces. It takes a great deal of force to cause a dislocation. For this reason, there are usually accompanying fractures of the radial head and coranoid process.

Approximately 90% of elbow dislocations occur posteriorly from a FOOSH-type injury. The other 10% of elbow dislocations may be anterior, divergent, medial, or lateral. Anterior dislocations usually occur from a direct blow to the posterior aspect of a flexed elbow and are commonly associated with brachial artery and median nerve injury. Divergent dislocations are extremely rare and caused by high-energy trauma to the elbow. Medial and lateral dislocations occur when the humerus is displaced either medially or laterally. See Figure 7.32 for an example of an elbow dislocation.

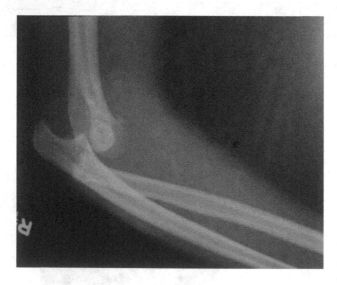

FIGURE 7.32 Elbow dislocation.
Courtesy of Theresa M. Campo.

Nurse maid's elbow is not a dislocation but a radial head subluxation. Nurse maid's elbow can occur between the ages of 1 to 5 years of age but most commonly occurs in the child between 2 and 3 years of age. The annular ligament becomes torn from the radial head during a sudden pull on the forearm with the arm extended and minimally pronated. The torn annular ligament then slips between the radial head and the capetellum. This injury does not require medical imaging with a plain radiograph unless the mechanism is of a direct blow or other traumatic event. Ultrasound is being used to identify nurse maid's elbow and confirm reduction of the annular ligament. However, clinical correlation with use of the arm again, following closed reduction, is typically confirmatory.

Wrist

Lunate and perilunate dislocations occur most frequently from a FOOSH but may also occur from a direct blow to the palm of the hand, causing dorsiflexion and ulnar deviation. Perilunate dislocations occur two to three times more frequently than lunate dislocations. Lunate dislocations occur when the lunate displaces volarly and rotates up to 90° from both the capitate and radius. Lunate dislocations are best seen in the lateral view with typical radius—lunate—capitate lines of the bones rotating medially and distally (Figure 7.33). Perilunate dislocations occur when the capitate is displaced from the lunate, most commonly toward the dorsal surface. Perilunate dislocations are also best visualized on the lateral view with the lunate in proper alignment with the radius with accompanying capitate dislocation. The AP view shows crowding of the carpals with overlapping of the proximal and distal rows. Approximately 75% of perilunate dislocations have an associated scaphoid fracture (Figure 7.34).

Phalanges

Dislocation can occur at any of the phalangeal joints and are considered either simple or complex. In simple dislocations, there is no soft tissue entrapment within the joint. When soft tissue becomes entrapped in the joint, the dislocation is considered to be complex and reduction may be quite difficult. Dislocation of matacarpal phalangeal/interpharlangeal (MCP/IP) joints is described by the specific affected joint and the direction of the distal phalanx.

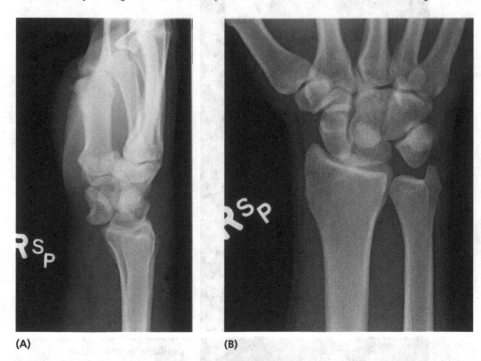

(A) (B)

FIGURE 7.33 (A) and (B) demonstrate a lunate dislocation.
Reprinted by permission of James Heilman, MD, Wikipedian, ER Department Head, East Kootenay Regional Hospital, Clinical Assistant Professor, Department of Emergency Medicine, University of British Columbia.

(A)

(B)

(C)

FIGURE 7.34 (A) through (C) demonstrate a perilunate dislocation.
Source: University of Virginia. Permission granted by the University of Virginia Department of Radiology and Medical Imaging.

It is important to note that any fracture or dislocation that is reduced should have a postreduction radiograph to confirm realignment and reduction. Postreduction images can also rule in or out an accompanying fracture that was not visible due to the dislocation. Depending on the extent and stability of the fracture and/or dislocation, the postreduction film may need to occur either before or after a splint or cast has been applied.

BONE LESIONS

When evaluating the bone structures, growths of a benign or malignant etiology may be identified. When evaluating a bony lesion on radiograph, one should consider if the margins are ill-defined, well-defined, or sclerotic. Next, consider the patient's age and, finally, where the lesion is located. Well-defined and sclerotic lesions in individuals younger than 40 years of age are usually benign with the exception of a well-defined chondrosarcoma, which occurs most often between the ages of 20 and 40 years. Ill-defined lytic lesions or any new bony lesions after the age of 40 years are highly suspicious for malignancy or metastasis and should have further evaluation (see Figure 7.35).

FIGURE 7.35 Ill-defined (A1) and well-defined lytic lesion great toe (A2); rim sclerotic lesion enchondroma right femur (B); and sclerotic lesions (C).

Courtesy of Dr. Douglas W. Parrillo; diagramming, Theresa M. Campo.

CONCLUSION

Falls and direct trauma are the most common causes of injury to the upper extremities. There are many terms used to identify types of fractures and dislocations. The important thing to remember is to clearly describe, using correct anatomical terminology, what is visualized on an image and not become overly concerned about the "proper name" of a fracture or dislocation. Proper identification of the bone, area of the bone, and type of fracture is all that is needed to discuss your findings with colleagues and radiologists. The ability to properly identify normal anatomical structures is paramount to understanding what you are visualizing on a radiograph and why. Always match the mechanism of injury with the findings themselves. If a mechanism does not match the findings, then suspicion for abuse is necessary and warranted. Keep looking at upper extremity films to improve your interpretation proficiency and confidence. Have fun!

RESOURCES

Au-Yong, I., Au-Yong, A., & Broderick, N. (2010). *On-call x-rays made easy.* Philadelphia, PA: Churchill Livingstone, Elsevier.

Campo, T., & Lafferty, K. A. (2016). *Essential procedures for emergency, urgent, and primary care settings.* New York, NY: Springer Publishing.

Daffner, R. H. (2014). Musculoskeletal imaging. In R. H. Daffner & M. S. Hartman (Eds.), *Clinical radiology: The essentials* (4th ed., pp. 353–429). Philadelphia, PA: Wolters Kluwer/Lippincott Williams & Wilkins.

Helms, C. A. (2012). Skeletal trauma. In W. E. Brant & C. A. Helms (Eds.), *Fundamentals of diagnostic radiology* (4th ed., pp. 1015–1042). Philadelphia, PA: Wolters Kluwer/Lippincott Williams & Wilkins.

Herring, W. (2016). *Learning radiology: Recognizing the basics* (3rd ed., pp. 240–253). Philadelphia, PA: Elsevier.

Kuntz, A. F., Lai, W. S., Norton, P. T., Yao, L. L., & Gay, S. B. Skeletal trauma. Retrieved from https://www.med-ed.virginia.edu/courses/rad/ext/index.html

Nunn, H., & Nunn, D. (n.d.). Norwich image interpretation course. Retrieved from http://www.imageinterpretation.co.uk

8

Basic Interpretation of Long Bone—Lower Extremity Radiographs

Radiographs of long bones, whether of the upper extremity or the lower extremity, are usually performed due to a traumatic injury. However, pain, swelling, and/or redness may also be indications for obtaining radiographs to rule out abnormal growth, infection, bursitis, or foreign body. Plain radiographs of long bones are beneficial in identifying fractures, subluxation, dislocation, and soft tissue swelling in traumatic injuries, but are also beneficial in identifying abnormal bone growths for nontraumatic signs and symptoms.

In this chapter, normal findings on the plain radiographs are discussed, as well as common findings in adults and children. When interpreting long-bone radiographs having the knowledge of normal anatomical structures is imperative. We discuss not only the anatomical structures on the radiographs but also normal alignment of joint structures and normal variants that may be seen on plain radiographs.

NORMAL

Before ordering any plain radiographs of long bones or joints, it is important to review some of the rules discussed in earlier chapters. When evaluating the lower extremity, it is important to not only assess the area of complaint but also to examine the joint above and below the affected area. For instance, if the patient complains of an injury to the shin, the radiological study should include the knee as well as the ankle. Routine studies should include a minimum of two views with most having three views, or more depending on the area in question.

Plain radiographs are excellent in identifying bony abnormalities such as fractures. Even though radiographs are not the best modality for evaluating soft tissue structures, such as cartilage, muscle, tendons, and ligaments, that make up a particular joint, plain films can identify changes within the alignment of the bones making up the joint and show edema that is inflammatory in nature, resulting from an occult bone fracture or from other causes of traumatic injury.

The lower extremity consists of the pelvis, hip, knee, ankle, metatarsal, and phalangeal joints, as well as the bones that make up these joints: the pelvic bones, femur, tibia, fibula, patella, tarsals, metatarsals, and phalanges. Each joint in each bone has a different appearance as well as function within the lower extremity. Any abnormalities can cause a loss of normal function and use of the lower extremity. As discussed in the previous chapter, there are five types of bones in the body; these can be seen in Table 7.1 of Chapter 7. When evaluating bone images, it is important to visualize the cortical margins in order to identify any abnormalities.

The ABCs of interpretation can be utilized for systematic assessment of the lower extremity. *A* is for *a*dequacy and *a*lignment. As stated in previous chapters, adequacy of the film is of the utmost importance when evaluating any radiographs. Knowledge of proper alignment allows the viewer to identify subtle abnormalities. Alignment refers to the bone itself and also with its orientation within the joint. *B* is for *b*ones and refers to the evaluation of all components of the bone in the respective study. Cortical margins and borders should be evaluated for any disruption or lack of continuity of that bone indicative of a fracture. Scan also for any abnormal growths or lesions, which may appear as densities or opacities on the radiograph image. *C*artilage and joints can be evaluated for abnormalities by visualizing the joint space. Loss of any joint space may be indicative of a crush injury or could be a sign of degenerative joint disease. Bulging or displacement of normal structures in the lower extremity may be indicative of a fracture or a joint effusion. *S*oft tissue can show signs of trauma through abnormal joint effusion or edema. Scan also for radiopaque foreign bodies within the bone and soft tissues.

DESCRIBING FRACTURES

A fracture or break to a bone or bones can happen from injury or pathology. Describe fractures using correct anatomical terminology when interpreting findings. Remember, fracture lines or patterns may be transverse, oblique, spiral, comminuted, impacted, avulsed, compressed, or depressed (Figure 8.1). Fractures may only involve one side of the bone, or both sides, or go completely through the bone itself.

Spiral   Displaced   Comminuted   Oblique   Transverse   Impacted

FIGURE 8.1 Fracture lines or patterns.
Drawing by Ocean City High School student.

Fractures may affect a single bone, may be noted in multiple bones, or there may be multiple fractures in the same bone but in different areas. Bone fragments may also be displaced or nondisplaced. When a bone fragment is 100% displaced, there is shortening along with overlapping of the bone fragments, referred to as a bayonet deformity (Figure 8.2). When bone fragments are out of alignment with each other, they are considered to be angulated. Angulation is the angle between the longitudinal axis of the main fracture fragment with that of the other fragment. Significant angulation requires reduction and realignment of the bone fragments for proper healing. If a fracture line enters into the joint space, it is referred to as an intra-articular fracture (Figure 8.3).

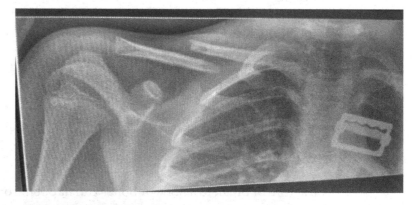

FIGURE 8.2 Bayonet deformity.
Courtesy of Dr. David Begleiter.

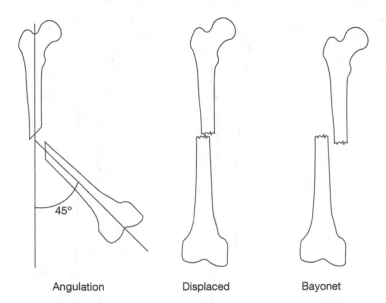

45°

Angulation   Displaced   Bayonet

FIGURE 8.3 Angulation, displacement, and bayonet deformity.
Drawing by Ocean City High School student.

A stress fracture can occur with repetitive loading beyond the bone's tolerance. An avulsion fracture occurs when there is a forcible muscular contraction affecting the tendinous attachment and a piece of bone is pulled off of the main structure.

PEDIATRIC CONSIDERATIONS

Consideration needs to be given with the pediatric patient. Pediatric bones are more fibrous and less crystalline (calcified) than adult bones. They are enclosed in a sheet of strong fibrous periosteum and have epiphyseal growth plates, which are a zone of weakness. Children tend to have incomplete fractures such as a greenstick fracture or torus fracture because the bone ends do not separate as in adults; this is due to the strong periosteal sleeve. The most common types of fractures in the pediatric patient are elastic deformation, bowing deformation, torus or buckle fracture, greenstick fracture, Salter–Harris fracture, stress injury, and avulsion injury (Figure 8.4).

Pediatric bones have epiphyseal growth plates that allow the bones to grow until they are mature adult bones. When a fracture occurs within or around the growth plate, it can complicate the healing process. Growth disturbances can be expected and the potential for loss of long bones may occur. However, current literature demonstrates that the loss of length after a fracture of a long bone tends to be made up in 1 to 2 years after the injury by overgrowth. The epiphyseal growth plate is a zone of weakness, which

Normal   Torus   Greenstick

FIGURE 8.4 Pediatric fracture.
Drawing by Ocean City High School student.

can make fracture, separation, and slipping of the growth plate more common in the pediatric patient.

There are five types of fractures that make up the Salter–Harris classification. The types of fractures are based on abnormalities involving the metaphysis, epiphysis, and/or diaphysis. A Salter I fracture is a separation of the growth plate without involvement of the metaphysis or the epiphysis. A Salter II fracture occurs across the growth plate but with a small fragment of metaphysis remaining attached to the epiphysis. A fracture across the growth plate with extension of the fracture line across the epiphysis is known as a Salter III fracture. When the fracture line traverses the epiphysis and part of the metaphysis, this is known as a Salter IV fracture. Finally, when there is damage to both the epiphysis and the metaphysis from a crush injury, this is known as a Salter V fracture. As you will notice, the severity of the injury increases with the designating number of the Salter–Harris fracture (see Figure 8.5). An easy mnemonic to remember the Salter classification is SALTR. *s* refers to a *slip* as in a Salter I, *a* refers to the fracture noted *above* or proximal to the epiphyseal plate, *l* refers to a fracture be*low* or distal to the epiphyseal plate, *t* is a fracture line extending *through* the epiphyseal plate including both the epiphysis and metaphysis, and *r* refers to *crush*.

FIGURE 8.5 Five types of Salter–Harris fractures.
Drawing by Ocean City High School student.

ABNORMALITIES OF THE LOWER EXTREMITY

Pelvis

The pelvis is composed of eight bones that make up three bone rings. The eight bones are the ilium (2), ischium (2), pubis (2), sacrum, and coccyx. There is one main ring that is made up of the sacroiliac joints and the symphysis pubis and two smaller rings made up of the pubis and ischial bones (see Figure 8.6). When imaging the pelvis, order an anterior–posterior (AP) view. When obtaining a pelvic image, it is important that the femurs are internally rotated on the AP view for visualization of the femoral neck. However, anterior and posterior oblique views can also be done since a true lateral is of no benefit. Additional views for further evaluation of the pelvis include the frog leg or frog lateral view.

FIGURE 8.6 Pelvic anatomy.
Source: Gray (1918).

Evaluating plain films of the pelvis and hips can be diagnostically challenging and may require CT scanning to further evaluate for occult fractures, identify complex fractures, or determine the degree of displacement and soft tissue injury. It is important to identify fractures and soft tissue abnormalities in the pelvis due to the potential for hemorrhage that may lead to death.

When scanning a pelvic radiograph, look for alignment within the joints, symmetry, cortical breaks, and joint spaces (sacroiliac, hip, symphysis pubis). It is important to see all aspects of the pelvis including the main ring, the two small rings, two sacroiliac joints, symphysis pubis, sacral foramina, and the acetabular region (Figure 8.7). When looking at the pelvic image, you want to ensure that the ilium and ischium are symmetrical and the main ring is circular with smooth borders. Envision that the ilium are ears, the main ring a face, and the ischium make up a bow tie. As long as all the parts are symmetrical and clear you should have a normal radiograph (Figure 8.8).

FIGURE 8.7 Normal pelvic radiograph.
Courtesy of Dr. David Begleiter.

FIGURE 8.8 Envisioning symmetry of the ilium and ischium and smooth borders of the main ring.
Courtesy of Dr. David Begleiter; diagramming, Theresa M. Campo.

When evaluating alignment, you should note Shenton's line, which is a curved line formed by the top of the obturator foramina in the inner side of the neck of the femur (Figure 8.9). This is used to determine the relationship of the head of the femur with the acetabulum. If this line is broken or is disrupted, then fracture or congenital luxation should be suspected. The bones and joints of the pelvis need to be evaluated for normal structure and joint space. The inner and outer cortices of the main ring as well as the formation of the obturator foramina of the two small rings need to be evaluated for disruption in the bone cortex. Scan the alignment of the superior surfaces of the pubic bone body of the symphysis pubis, which also needs to be evaluated. The sacral foramina should be evaluated for any disruption of the smooth arcuate lines, indicating a fracture, and the arcs should be compared. The acetabular region should be evaluated for any gross abnormalities; if any are identified, views of the hip should also be obtained for further evaluation. See Figure 8.10 for marked structures.

FIGURE 8.9 Shenton's line.
Courtesy of Dr. David Begleiter; diagramming, Theresa M. Campo.

FIGURE 8.10 Pelvic radiograph with marking of structures.
Courtesy of Dr. David Begleiter; diagramming, Theresa M. Campo.

Assess the symphysis pubis for alignment of the superior surfaces of the pubic bone body. The symphysis pubis width can be up to 10 mm in children but should never be more than 5 mm in adults. The superior cortices of the superior pubic rami should be in alignment. The ischial-pubic synchondrosis may present as being irregular and asymmetrical during development until approximately the age of 12 years old. The sacroiliac joints may appear normally wide in adolescents, but in adults, they should not be more than 2 to 4 mm in width.

Disruptions in the bone cortex and joint space of the pelvis may not only occur on one side but may occur in another area due to the nature of the pelvis and its three bone rings. If the main pelvic ring is broken into two areas, then it is considered to be unstable with the risk of hemorrhage and shock. This injury may also be accompanied by bladder rupture and urethral injury, requiring careful evaluation of the urethra with a retrograde urethrogram prior to any urinary catheterization. Avulsion injuries can be common in the adolescent age group and can be easily missed. Frequent sites for avulsion injuries are the anterior superior iliac spine, anterior inferior iliac spine, and the ischial tuberosity. Complex fractures should be considered, particularly when the sacrum or iliac wing is involved, which were caused by increased force.

Pelvic Fractures

A straddle injury can cause force against the perineum, resulting in fracture of the pubic rami bilaterally with the central fragment being displaced superiorly. This may be accompanied by an acetabulum fracture and associated with dislocation, which is usually posterior.

Vertical shearing may result in a vertical, unilateral fracture of the pelvic rami with a vertical fracture of the sacral foramina on the same side. This may cause disruption of the sacroiliac joints and possibly fracture to the ilium, paralleling the sacroiliac joint.

A Malgaigne fracture occurs when there is an articular or para-articular fracture of the sacroiliac joint and ipsilateral ischiopubic rami. Clinically, you will observe shortening of the ipsilateral lower extremity (see Figure 8.11).

Avulsion fractures can also occur within the pelvis and be easily missed. Common areas of avulsion injury are the inferior and superior anterior iliac spines and the ischial tuberosity. These injuries are usually sport related and seen in sprinters, gymnasts, cheerleaders, and track and field athletes (sprinters, jumpers, etc.). These injuries are usually caused by the sudden strong contraction of large muscles.

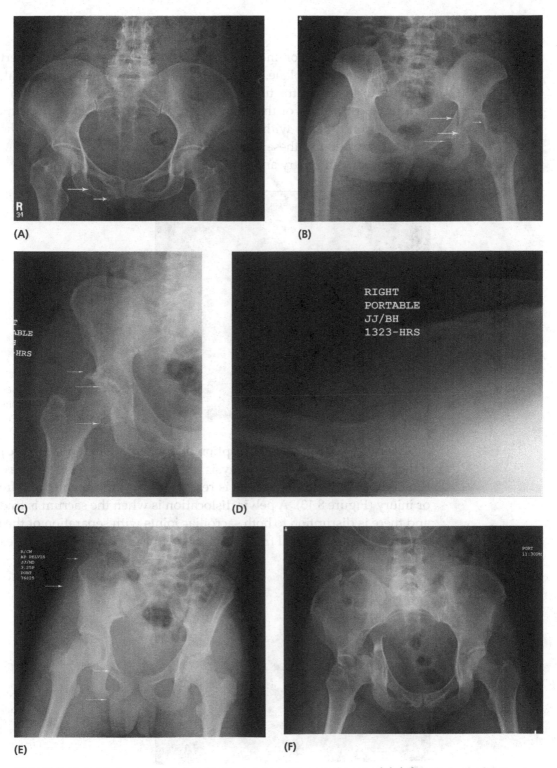

FIGURE 8.11 Pelvic fractures. Pelvic fracture right ischium and ramus (A); left acetabular fracture (B); comminuted right acetabular fracture (C); comminuted right acetabular fracture (D); multiple fractures including alar fx (E); and pelvic fracture with displacement (F).

Courtesy of Dr. Douglas W. Parrillo; diagramming, Theresa M. Campo.

Sacral Fracture

Sacral fractures are commonly missed and usually occur either vertically or in the transverse plane. Bowel gas may obscure the sacrum, making it difficult to visualize fractures. Sacral fractures may co-occur with pelvic injuries and fractures or they may occur on their own. Examination of the sacrum should begin with the arcuate lines bilaterally to see if they are intact. Disruption of these lines is indicative of a fracture. See Figure 8.12 regarding the symmetry and asymmetry of arcuate lines.

FIGURE 8.12 Arcuate lines.
Courtesy of Dr. David Begleiter; diagramming, Theresa M. Campo.

Anterior force can cause disruption of one or both of the sacroiliac joints. If there is widening of the symphysis pubis greater than 5 mm with external rotation of the hemi pelvis, this is referred to as the "open book" fracture or injury (Figure 8.13). A pelvic dislocation is when the sacrum is fractured and there is disruption to both sacroiliac joints with separation of the pubis symphysis. Occult sacral fractures may be present if there is fracture of the L5 transverse process.

FIGURE 8.13 "Open book" fracture.
Courtesy of Dr. Douglas W. Parrillo.

Hip

The hip is composed of the acetabulum and the femoral head, the along with ligaments, the joint capsule, and articular cartilage. When evaluating the hip, AP, lateral, and oblique views are necessary. A one-view pelvis should always be included in the evaluation of the hip (Figure 8.14). The AP view of the hip and pelvis should have the hips internally rotated for full visualization of the femoral neck. Ensure that all views fit the adequacy criteria and evaluate the alignment of the bones that make up the hip joint. You will need to evaluate the bone margins for any abnormalities and evaluate the joint itself for signs of effusion or secondary signs of a possible occult fracture. Finally, evaluate soft tissue for any foreign bodies, gas collection, or other abnormalities (see Figure 8.15). If x-rays of the hip and pelvis are obtained and show no signs of fracture, it is important to make sure that the patient is able to walk on his or her own; if not, a CT scan may be necessary to rule out an occult fracture. Fractures of the acetabulum may be difficult to identify but are of utmost importance.

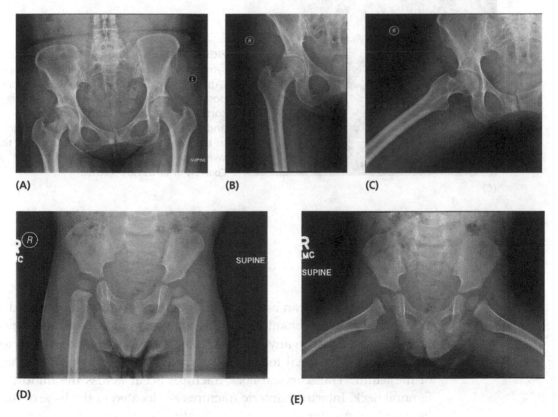

(A)   (B)   (C)

(D)   (E)

FIGURE 8.14 Normal adult pelvic image (A); normal adult hip images (B and C); and normal pediatric hip images (D and E).
Courtesy of Dr. David Begleiter.

(A)

(B)

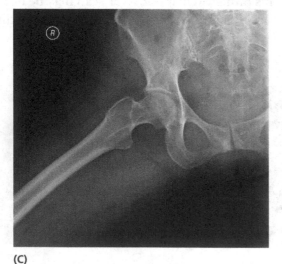

(C)

FIGURE 8.15 Evaluation of the pelvis image for symmetry and breaks in the lines of the pelvis (A); evaluation of the hip image, anterior–posterior view, for alignment of the bony cortex joint space and soft tissue swelling (B); and evaluation of the hip image for alignment of the bony cortex, joint space, and soft tissue swelling (C).
Courtesy of Dr. David Begleiter.

Femur

The proximal femur can be divided into five areas: the femoral head, neck, greater and lesser trochanter, and the proximal femoral shaft (Figure 8.16). Fractures can occur in any of these areas; therefore, it is important to note the location. Subcapital femoral neck fractures occur just below the head of the femur. Transcervical neck fractures occur across the middle of the femoral neck. Intertrochanteric fractures are located at the base of the neck between the greater and lesser trochanter. Fractures can also occur along the greater trochanter, lesser trochanter, or below in the subtrochanteric region (see Figure 8.17).

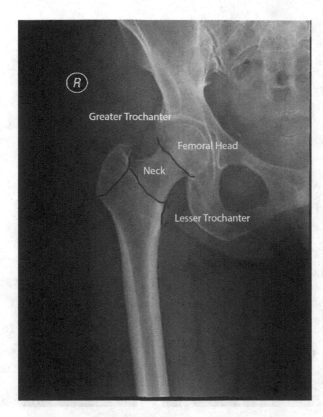

FIGURE 8.16 Areas of the proximal femur.
Courtesy of Dr. David Begleiter; diagramming, Theresa M. Campo.

(A)

FIGURE 8.17 Different fracture areas of the proximal femur. Subcapital fracture proximal femur (A).

(continued)

(B)

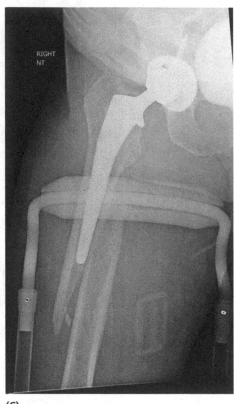

(C)

FIGURE 8.17 (*continued*) Proximal femur fracture (note the traction splint) (B and C). Courtesy of Dr. Douglas W. Parrillo.

Most commonly, subcapital fractures are impacted or displaced and may be complete or incomplete. They most commonly result from postmenopausal osteoporosis in women. Avascular necrosis of the femoral head may occur in approximately 20% to 30% of subcapital fractures secondary to the disruption or impingement of the femoral complex arteries. Intertrochanteric femoral fractures generally occur in the older adults and are more frequent than subcapital in this aging population.

The femur also has the potential to dislocate either anterior or posterior to the acetabulum. The majority of dislocations occur posteriorly approximately 90% of the time. The most common mechanism causing a posterior dislocation is a high-energy trauma, such as when the knees impact a dashboard during a motor vehicle accident. Assess for a possible posterior rim acetabular fracture, which may accompany a dislocation. The femoral head sits lateral and superior to the acetabulum with internal rotation and abduction of the femur. The femoral head may appear smaller on the radiographic image secondary to magnification (see Figure 8.18).

FIGURE 8.18 Hip dislocation.
Reprinted by permission of James Heilman, MD,
Wikipedian, ER Department Head, East Kootenay
Regional Hospital, Clinical Assistant Professor,
Department of Emergency Medicine, University of
British Columbia.

Avascular necrosis, also known as osteonecrosis, can be a painful weight-bearing condition that can occur from trauma, prolonged corticosteroid use, alcohol abuse, chemotherapy, sickle-cell disease, or history of a diving and nitrogen toxicity type injury. Avascular necrosis occurs from lack of blood supply to the femoral head resulting in bone death (see Figure 8.19).

FIGURE 8.19 Avascular necrosis (AVN). Note loss
of integrity bony cortex (top image).
Reprinted with permission from Medscape Drugs &
Diseases (http://emedicine.medscape.com), 2016.
Available at http://emedicine.medscape.com/
article/386808-overview

Midshaft femur fractures can occur anywhere along the femoral shaft and may be transverse, oblique, spiral, or comminuted. It can take a great deal of force to cause a fracture in the femur so it is important to ascertain that the mechanism matches the finding on the radiograph. Distal fractures can involve either the medial or lateral condyle of the femur leading up into the shaft (Figure 8.20). These can be complex injuries with a lot of soft tissue swelling and the potential for a large volume blood loss.

FIGURE 8.20 Medial and lateral condyle fractures. Midshaft femur fracture (A, B, and C).

(continued)

(E)   (F)

FIGURE 8.20 (*continued*) Distal femur fracture (D, E, and F). Courtesy of Dr. Douglas W. Parrillo.

In children, abnormalities of the hip joint or femur can occur. A slipped femoral capital epiphysis (SFCE) is a Salter I fracture and commonly occurs in overweight children and adolescent boys older than the age of 8 years. It can occur either unilaterally or bilaterally and may be associated with minor trauma. A SFCE presents on a plain film as widening of the epiphyseal plate of the proximal femur. Obtaining a frog leg view may make it easier to identify medial slipping of the epiphyseal plate much better than could be visualized on the AP view. To identify this abnormality, draw a line along the lateral femoral neck. If it is not congruent and does not intersect the femoral epiphysis, then it may indicate medial slipping of the epiphyseal plate. See Figure 8.21 demonstrating a SFCE and the lines demonstrating the abnormality.

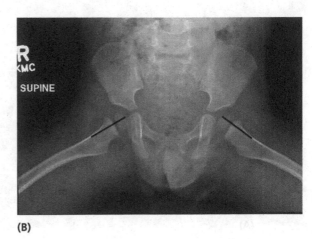

(A)   (B)

FIGURE 8.21 (A) and (B) demonstrate a normal adult hip.

(C)

FIGURE 8.21 (*continued*) Slipped capital epiphysis (note the malalignment of the epiphysis and metaphysis) (C)
Courtesy of Dr. Douglas W. Parrillo; diagramming, Theresa M. Campo.

Osteochondritis can occur in numerous places in the body and is labeled based on the area where it is found. Legg–Calve–Perthes disease denotes an osteochondritis occurring at the femoral head. This most commonly occurs in boys younger than the age of 8. On a plain film, the femoral head will appear to have a patchy sclerotic and flattened articular surface resulting from avascular necrosis (Figure 8.22).

(A)

(B)

FIGURE 8.22 Legg–Calve–Perthes disease. Note the abnormality of the femoral head (A, B, and C).

(*continued*)

FIGURE 8.22 (*continued*) Courtesy of Dr. Douglas W. Parrillo.

(C)

Knee

The knee is a large complex joint with three articulations: medial tibial femoral, lateral tibial femoral, and patellofemoral. Stability of the knee is provided by four ligaments: the medial, lateral collateral, anterior, and posterior cruciate ligaments. Evaluation of the knee should include an AP, lateral, and two oblique views (Figure 8.23). An additional image that may be useful in evaluating patellar fractures is the sunrise view, also referred to as a skyline view (Figure 8.24).

(A)

(B)

FIGURE 8.23 Five views of knee. Normal adult knee images (A and B).

(*continued*)

FIGURE 8.23 (*continued*)
Normal pediatric images (C, D, and E).
Courtesy of Dr. David Begleiter

Injuries to the knee are common due to the complexity of the joint. They most commonly involve soft tissue and cartilaginous structures. Radiographs are useful in identifying fractures as well as effusion. However, an MRI is the best modality for evaluating this complex joint.

Knee fractures can be caused by either a direct blow or from a violent contraction of the quadricep muscle. It is best to obtain a sunrise view to evaluate for occult and overt fracture of the patella. Patellar fractures may be vertical, horizontal, or comminuted. If a transverse fracture of the patella is suspected or visualized in the AP view, then you should not perform a sunrise view. Manipulation of the knee can cause displacement. A transverse avulsion patellar fracture can result from violent contraction of the quadricep muscle, which occurs with sports activities. Transverse avulsion fractures are more common than longitudinal or comminuted patellar fractures. A bipartite patella can be differentiated from an acute

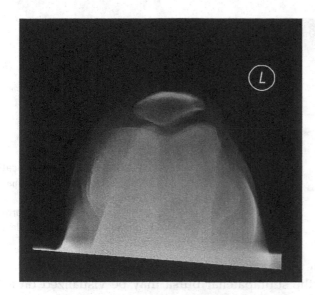

FIGURE 8.24 Sunrise view.
Courtesy of Dr. David Begleiter.

fracture by looking at the abnormality. It is important to differentiate a bipartite patella from a true acute fracture (Figure 8.25). The bipartite patella will have round margins that don't easily fit together. However, the fracture will look like a piece of a puzzle and can be put together visually (Figure 8.25).

FIGURE 8.25 Bipartite. Note well-corticated area in circles.
Courtesy of Heller Hoff (2016)/Wikipedia Commons; diagramming, Theresa M. Campo.

True dislocations of the knee are rare but usually occur in an anterior translation of the tibia on the femur. Anterior translation is when the tibia displaces anterior to the femur. In the case of a true dislocation, consideration of a popliteal artery and/or nerve injury as well as multiple ligamentous tears should be entertained. This usually occurs from an acute injury and can be diagnosed easily even before a radiograph is obtained (see Figure 8.26).

FIGURE 8.26 Knee dislocation. *Source:* University of Virginia. Permission granted by the University of Virginia Department of Radiology and Medical Imaging.

Inflammation of the suprapatellar bursa may be visualized on a knee radiographic study. A fat pad in the anterior and posterior compartments of the suprapatellar bursa is located posterior to the quadricep tendon in the joint capsule. This corresponding area of the fat pad should normally measure less than 5 mm. However, the fat pad can expand from an effusion indicative of a soft tissue injury. Additionally, intra-articular fractures may also cause leakage of blood and bone marrow into the joint space, distending the bursa and enlarging the fat pad. Fat lying on top of the fluid is seen radiographically as a fluid–fluid line or density on the lateral view. This is highly indicative of an intra-articular fracture even if one is not visualized in the images of the study (see Figure 8.27).

FIGURE 8.27 Knee effusion. Courtesy of Dr. Douglas W. Parrillo.

Tibia

The tibia plateau can be divided into the lateral and medial aspect (Figure 8.28). Fractures to the tibial plateau are commonly labeled as "fender" or "bumper" fractures because they can be caused by a motor vehicle striking a person's leg. Tibial plateau fractures commonly occur on the lateral aspect and may be associated with an anterior cruciate ligament (ACL), medial cruciate ligament (MCL), or medial meniscus injury from valgus stress placed on the knee. It is important to look closely at the tibial plateau because it may be difficult to visualize a fracture if it is not depressed or impacted. Look closely for a lucent fracture line with increased density, denoting impaction or depression. It is also important to draw a perpendicular line at the most lateral margin of the femoral condyle and medial cortex of the fibula. These areas should be in alignment and there should not be more than 5 mm of the condyle located laterally (see Figures 8.29 and 8.30).

FIGURE 8.28 Medial and lateral aspect tibia plateau.
Courtesy of Dr. David Begleiter; diagramming, Theresa M. Campo.

FIGURE 8.29 Medial and lateral lines.
Courtesy of Dr. David Begleiter; diagramming, Theresa M. Campo.

(A)

(B)

(C)

(D)

FIGURE 8.30 (A) through (D) demonstrate tibial plateau fractures.

(continued)

(E)

(F)

(G)

FIGURE 8.30 (*continued*) Lateral tibial plateau fractures (E through G).
Courtesy of Dr. Douglas W. Parrillo and University of Virginia. Permission granted by the University of Virginia Department of Radiology and Medical Imaging.

A Segond fracture is an avulsion of the lateral aspect of the tibial plateau at the attachment of the lateral capsule (Figure 8.31). This injury results from varus stress with internal rotation of the leg, with the knee in a flexed position putting excess tension on the lateral capsule and its associated ligaments. This mechanism may also cause an accompanying ACL tear.

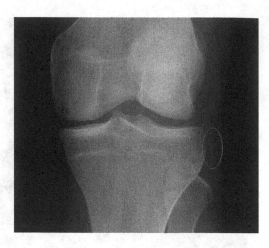

FIGURE 8.31 Segond fracture.
Courtesy of Ellisbjohns (2009)/Wikipedia Commons.

Midshaft fractures of the tibia may occur solely or with an accompanying fibula fracture, depending on the mechanism of injury and the force allotted to cause the fracture. Fractures may occur anywhere along the shaft of the tibia and should be matched with the mechanism of injury to rule out abuse as the cause of injury.

An avulsion of the lateral margin of the distal tibia is known as a Tillaux fracture (Figure 8.32). The mechanism of this injury is abduction and external rotation of the leg. A fracture line vertically extending from the distal articular surface in an upward direction to the lateral cortex of the tibia will be seen on a plain film. Surgery for this injury may be required if there is lateral displacement of the fracture fragments distal to the articular surface. Otherwise, conservative treatment is usually indicated if no displacement is involved.

FIGURE 8.32 Tillaux fracture.
Source: University of Virginia. Permission granted by the University of Virginia Department of Radiology and Medical Imaging.

Fibula

Proximal fibula fractures of the head and neck may be associated with tibial plateau fractures or ligamentous injuries to the cruciate or collateral ligaments of the knee. The Maisonneuve fracture occurs when there is strong eversion of the ankle, causing a fracture to the proximal half of the fibula accompanied by fracture of the medial malleolus of the distal tibia and disruption of the tibiofibular syndesmosis (complete tear may occur) (see Figure 8.33).

FIGURE 8.33 Maisonneuve fracture.
Courtesy of Dr. Douglas W. Parrillo.

Midshaft fractures of the fibula may occur in conjunction with a midshaft tibia fracture. When examining a plain film of the tibia and fibula, visually trace the margins of both bones in their entirety, looking for any disruptions, lucencies, or densities indicative of multiple fractures.

Osteochondritis of the anterior tibial tuberosity, also known as Osgood Schlatter's disease, occurs in adolescents. This often painful, inflammatory condition usually occurs from repeated trauma to a normal growth zone and ossification center at the tibial tuberosity. This condition can present on a radiographic image with a wide variety of normal variance and may be mistaken for an avulsion fracture (Figure 8.34).

FIGURE 8.34 Osgood Schlatter disease. Reprinted by permission of James Heilman, MD, Wikipedian, ER Department Head, East Kootenay Regional Hospital, Clinical Assistant Professor, Department of Emergency Medicine, University of British Columbia.

Ankle

The ankle consists of articulations between the three structures of the tibia, fibula, and talus. These three bones, along with the medial and lateral collateral ligaments and interosseous ligament, provide stability to the ankle joint (Figure 8.35). Obtaining AP, lateral, and mortise views are necessary for fully evaluating the ankle. The AP view will demonstrate a longer lateral malleolus than the medial malleolus (Figure 8.36A). The mortise view requires an oblique view at 20° to 30° of internal rotation that allows for alignment of the lateral and medial malleoli (Figure 8.36B). Bohler's angle is formed by drawing two lines. The first is drawn tangent to the superior aspect of the calcaneus and the second is drawn tangent to the inferior aspect of calcaneus. A normal Bohler's angle should be between 20° and 40°. The lateral view should show open collimation and include the calcaneus, base of the fifth metatarsal, and the dorsal surface of the talus and navicular bone (Figure 8.36C).

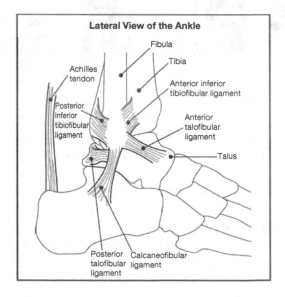

FIGURE 8.35 Ankle anatomy.
Source: https://en.wikipedia.org/wiki/Ankle

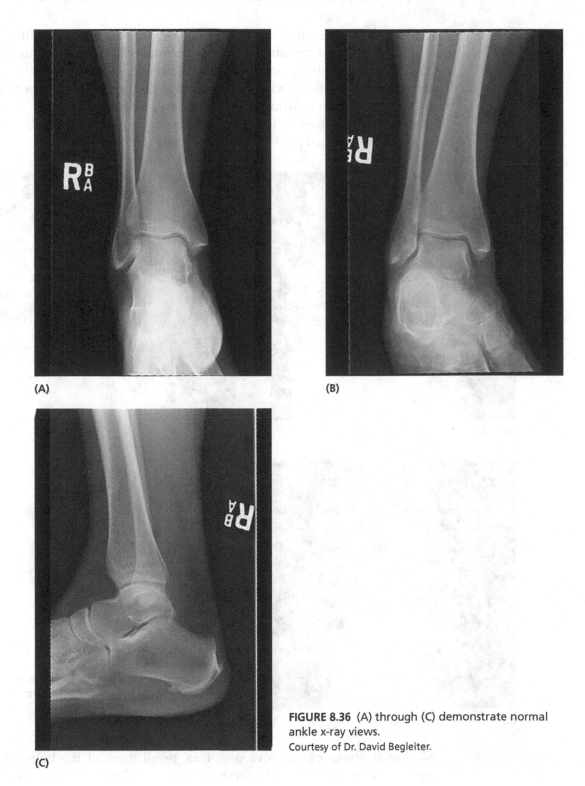

FIGURE 8.36 (A) through (C) demonstrate normal ankle x-ray views.
Courtesy of Dr. David Begleiter.

Trauma to the ankle can result from either inversion or eversion injury, direct blow, extreme dorsiflexion or plantar flexion, or a combination of all of these. Ligament damage can occur with or without an effusion.

Ligamentous injuries most commonly occur from inversion, resulting in soft tissue swelling of the lateral aspect of the ankle that may be visualized on the radiograph without an accompanied fracture. Joint effusion can also occur without a fracture and may be accompanied by soft tissue swelling from the injury. Joint effusions are most often seen in the anterior aspect of the ankle where fluid accumulates, appearing as a semicircular density anterior to the talotibial joint on the lateral view (Figure 8.37).

(A)

(B)

(C)

FIGURE 8.37 (A) through (C) demonstrate soft tissue swelling of the ankle.
Source: University of Virginia. Permission granted by the University of Virginia Department of Radiology and Medical Imaging.

Mortise fractures can involve one, two, or all three of the bones that comprise the ankle. The ankle forms a ring; therefore, if you identify a displaced fracture, be suspicious of another fracture. Ligamentous injuries of the medial collateral and lateral collateral ligaments may also rupture. If rupture occurs, there may be an accompanying avulsion fracture as well as soft tissue swelling. Ligamentous rupture can be assessed by evaluating at approximately 1 cm proximal to the tibial plafond distribution found between the tibia and fibula and should not measure more than 6 mm (Figure 8.38).

FIGURE 8.38 Ankle effusion.
Source: University of Virginia. Permission granted by the University of Virginia Department of Radiology and Medical Imaging.

When assessing for ankle fractures, scan the medial, lateral, and posterior malleolus and talus for any disruption, avulsion, or displacement. If an isolated distal fibula fracture or lateral malleolus fracture is identified, it is important to focus on the posterior aspect for an accompanying fracture. If there is displacement of the fracture of the medial malleolus or posterior malleolus, then a full-length tibia/fibula study is necessary to assess for an accompanying fracture. It is also important to identify widening of the medial joint space.

There are also accessory ossicles, which are unfused secondary ossification centers within the ankle. These ossicles will appear well corticated on imaging. An os subfibulare can be seen distal to the tip of the lateral malleolus. An os subtibiale can be seen distal to the tip of the medial malleolus and an os trigonum is located posterior to the talus (see Figure 8.39).

Foot

The foot can be divided into three regions: the forefoot, midfoot, and hindfoot.

The hindfoot consists of the talus and calcaneus. The midfoot includes the navicular, cuboid, and three cuneiforms. The metatarsals and phalanges make up the forefoot. When imaging the foot, obtaining AP, lateral, and oblique views (Figure 8.40) with an occasional tangential film will aid in identifying abnormalities of the three regions of the foot. Fractures occur more often than dislocations. However, fractures and dislocations can occur simultaneously.

(B)

FIGURE 8.39 Images (A) and (B) demonstrate the unfused secondary ossification centers.

Courtesy of Dr. David Begleiter; diagramming, Theresa M. Campo.

(A)

(A)

(B)

FIGURE 8.40 (A) through (C) are three views of the foot.

(continued)

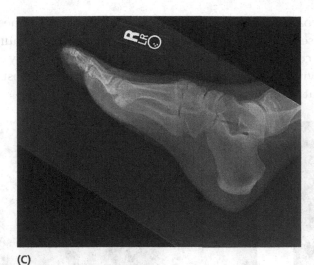

FIGURE 8.40 (*continued*)
Courtesy of Dr. David Begleiter.

(C)

Talus

The body of the talus includes the talar dome, which is divided into the medial and lateral aspects (Figure 8.41). Fractures to the body of the talus often involve the medial and lateral aspect of the talar dome. Fractures to the talar neck can place a person at high risk for developing avascular necrosis. Inversion injuries of the ankle can cause avulsion fractures of the talus.

FIGURE 8.41 Medial and lateral aspect of the talar dome.
Courtesy of Dr. David Begleiter; diagramming, Theresa M. Campo.

A talo-calcaneal coalition is defined as a union of one or more bones that are not normally fused. This is very rare and is not caused by a traumatic injury. Patients will complain of deep foot pain that is aggravated by activity and gets better with rest. The radiographic image will reveal closure of the subtalar joint that may be partial or complete (Figure 8.42).

(A)   **(B)**

FIGURE 8.42 (A) and (B) demonstrate talo-calcaneal coalition.
Source: University of Virginia. Permission granted by the University of Virginia Department of Radiology and Medical Imaging.

Calcaneus

Calcaneal fractures most commonly occur from a fall from heights. They are identified by a Bohler's angle that is less than 20°. However, a compression fracture cannot be excluded if the Bohler's angle is within normal limits. Because of the mechanism of injury, these fractures are commonly associated with spinal compression fractures, femoral neck fractures, and tibial plateau fractures. If a calcaneal fracture or fractures are identified, it is important to order imaging of the hips and spine. Evaluation of the subtalar joint is also necessary for identifying calcaneal fracture on imaging. Stress fractures of the calcaneus can also occur and are most commonly seen in runners and older adults. Figure 8.43 demonstrates various calcaneal fractures found on radiograph.

Tarsals

The midfoot consists of the tarsal bones of the foot: the navicular, cuboid, and the three cuneiforms (Figure 8.44). Fractures can occur in any of these bones and should be evaluated on all images (Figure 8.45).

FIGURE 8.43 (A) through (E) demonstrate various calcaneal fractures seen on a radiograph.
Source: University of Virginia. Permission granted by the University of Virginia Department of Radiology and Medical Imaging.

FIGURE 8.44 Images (A) and (B) show the bones of the foot
Courtesy of Dr. Keith Lafferty; diagramming, Theresa M. Campo.

FIGURE 8.45 (A) through (C) demonstrate fractures of the tarsal bones.
Reprinted by permission of James Heilman, MD, Wikipedian, ER Department Head, East Kootenay Regional Hospital, Clinical Assistant Professor, Department of Emergency Medicine, University of British Columbia.

Metatarsals

The five metatarsals are part of the forefoot. Fracture to the base of the fifth metatarsal that is at least 1.5 cm distal to the metatarsal styloid is known as a Jones fracture (Figure 8.46). The Jones fracture is commonly confused with an unfused apophysis and avulsion fracture of the metatarsal tuberosity at the insertion of the peroneus brevis tendon. A Jones fracture is not an

FIGURE 8.46 Images (A) through (D) demonstrate the Jones fracture.
Courtesy of Dr. Douglas W. Parrillo.

avulsion injury. An unfused apophysis of the fifth metatarsal usually occurs in a lengthwise pattern and lies parallel to the long axis of the metatarsal (Figure 8.47). An avulsion fracture usually occurs from an inversion injury (running in heels), occurs at the metatarsal tuberosity at the insertion of the peroneus brevis tendon, or occurs from violent contraction with force.

A Lisfranc injury is a fracture with or without dislocation at the tarsometatarsal joint. This fracture may occur when riding a motorbike or mountain bike and getting the foot caught in the pedal clips or when jamming the foot from a fall down stairs. This fracture is named after Napoleon's surgeon saw this type of injury from soldiers being knocked off of horses with their foot still in the stirrup. The mechanism causes a traumatic dorsiflexion that may also involve rotation. Although an uncommon injury, it is important to consider traumatic foot injuries. A Lisfranc injury will cause loss of normal alignment at the base of the second metatarsal. There may also be a fracture to the base of the second metatarsal and loss of alignment at the third metatarsal (see Figure 8.48).

Midshaft fractures of the metatarsals may occur in a transverse oblique manner. They may occur in one metatarsal or in multiple metatarsals. It is important to note the displacement and angulation, which may affect the type of treatment (see Figure 8.49).

FIGURE 8.47 Unfused apophysis.
Courtesy of Theresa M. Campo.

FIGURE 8.48 Lisfranc injury.
Reprinted by permission of James Heilman, MD, Wikipedian, ER Department Head, East Kootenay Regional Hospital, Clinical Assistant Professor, Department of Emergency Medicine, University of British Columbia.

(A)

(B)

FIGURE 8.49 (A) and (B) demonstrate metatarsal fractures.
Courtesy of Dr. Douglas W. Parrillo.

Phalanges

The phalanges make up the other part of the forefoot. Fractures most commonly occur in the proximal phalanx but may occur in any phalanges. Fracture may occur in one phalanx or multiple phalanges. Dislocations are also common in the toes and may be accompanied by fractures (see Figure 8.50).

(A) (B)

(C) (D)

FIGURE 8.50 (A) through (D) demonstrate first distal phalanx fractures.
Courtesy of Kyle Deuter; diagramming, Theresa M. Campo.

CONCLUSION

The lower extremity consists of not only complex joints but also weight-bearing bones. Both of these can cause difficulty in identifying abnormalities of not only the bones but also the soft tissue, including cartilage, ligaments, and muscle, as well as joint effusions.

RESOURCES

Au-Yong, I., Au-Yong, A., & Broderick, N. (2010). *On-call x-rays made easy*. Philadelphia, PA: Churchill Livingstone, Elsevier.

Daffner, R. H. (2014). Musculoskeletal imaging. In R. H. Daffner & M. S. Hartman (Eds.), *Clinical radiology: The essentials* (4th ed., pp. 353–429). Philadelphia, PA: Wolters Kluwer/Lippincott Williams & Wilkins.

Gray, H. (1918). *Anatomy of the human body*. Henry Vandyke Cater (illustrator). Philadelphia, PA: Lea and Febiger Publishers. Retrieved from https:// en.wikipedia.org/wiki/Pelvis#/media/File:Gray241.png

Helms, C. A. (2012). Miscellaneous bone lesions. In W. E. Brant & C. A. Helms (Eds.), *Fundamentals of diagnostic radiology* (4th ed., pp. 1090–1097). Philadelphia, PA: Wolters Kluwer/Lippincott Williams & Wilkins.

Helms, C. A. (2012). Skeletal trauma. In W. E. Brant & C. A. Helms (Eds.), *Fundamentals of diagnostic radiology* (4th ed., pp. 1015–1042). Philadelphia, PA: Wolters Kluwer/Lippincott Williams & Wilkins.

Herring, W. (2016). *Learning radiology: Recognizing the basics* (3rd ed., pp. 240–253). Philadelphia, PA: Elsevier.

Kuntz, A. F., Lai, W. S., Norton, P. T., Yao, L. L., & Gay, S. B. (n.d.). Skeletal trauma. Retrieved from https://www.med-ed.virginia.edu/courses/rad/ext/index.html

UNIT IV

Interpretation of Spine Radiographs

Basic Interpretation of Cervical Spine Radiographs

Cervical spine imaging and interpretation of spinal radiographs can be challenging. Guidelines such as the National Emergency X-Radiography Utilization Study (NEXUS) criteria and Canadian C-Spine (cervical spine) Rules (CCR) provide evidence-based guidelines for determining whether medical imaging is necessary. The NEXUS criteria guidelines are based on five factors: focal neural deficit, presence of midline spine tenderness, altered level of consciousness, presence of intoxication, and a distracting injury. The CCR have three categories with an algorithmic approach to decision making for imaging. If they have any high-risk factors such as age older than 65 years, having a dangerous mechanism of injury, and/or presence of paresthesia, then spinal images are indicated. If the patient does not have any of these risk factors but has pain with examination of the cervical spine and gentle passive range of motion, then imaging is warranted. Finally, if no pain was elicited during the assessment, the patient is asked to actively rotate the neck; if any pain or limitation is noted, imaging is indicated.

The three views of the cervical spine radiographic study are the anterior–posterior (AP), lateral, and odontoid views (Figure 9.1). The first view is the lateral, performed before spinal immobilization is removed. An adequate lateral view must include all seven vertebrae from C1 to the top of T1, including the junction of C7–T1 (Figure 9.2). If the patient has a thick neck or if the soft tissue is hindering the adequacy of the view, then traction on the arms, pulling downward toward the feet, can be performed to enhance the view. If that

(A)

(B)

(C)

FIGURE 9.1 Anterior–posterior view
(A); lateral view (B); odontoid view (C).
Courtesy of Theresa M. Campo.

FIGURE 9.2 Normal lateral view including T1
and showing the C7–T1 junction.
Courtesy of Theresa M. Campo.

does not improve the adequacy of the view, then a swimmer's view may be obtained. In a swimmer's view, the patient places one arm over his or her head, which aids in viewing the entire cervical spine. Once an adequate lateral image is obtained and visualized and no abnormalities are identified, the view should be repeated after the cervical collar is removed. In the AP view, the patient's mouth is closed during imaging, whereas in the odontoid view the mouth is kept open, which provides the best image of C1 and C2 (Figure 9.3).

FIGURE 9.3 Odontoid view. Note: Open mouth allowing for visualization of C1 and C2.
Courtesy of Theresa M. Campo.

If pain is present and there are no signs of any abnormalities with the routine three views, then a flexion and extension view can be obtained (Figure 9.4). A CT scan is not mandatory for evaluating the cervical spine, but if there are any injuries questioned or suspected on plain radiographs then it should be considered. CT scanning may also be considered in the elderly patient to improve identification of fractures which may be difficult to appreciate with arthritic changes on plain films. If ligamentous injury, neurological deficits, or spinal canal involvement are either suspected or confirmed by plain radiographs, CT scan, or MRI of the cervical spine should be obtained since it is excellent at contrasting soft tissue.

FIGURE 9.4 Flexion view (A); extension view (B).
Courtesy of Dr. Douglas W. Parrillo.

(A)   (B)

NORMAL

When evaluating the cervical spine on plain radiographs, it is important to look at each view in its entirety; however, your approach may be slightly different from one image to the other with regards to the ABCs that we've been using throughout this text. We will talk about each view in detail with regards to visualizing normal and identifying abnormal findings.

Lateral View

The lateral view is best for detecting most abnormalities in the cervical spine radiographs. Before beginning interpretation of the lateral view, it is important to ensure *a*dequacy. The provider must be able to visualize from C1 down to at least the top of T1, including the C7–T1 junction (Figure 9.2). It is also important to identify that there is good penetration with contrast occurring between the bony structures and the soft tissue.

When assessing for *a*lignment, there are four anatomical lines that need to be evaluated. The first two lines should be drawn from the odontoid peg through to the top of T1 along the anterior margin and posterior margin of the vertebral bodies. The third line should be drawn along the spinolaminar junction and a fourth line should be along the posterior spinous processes. Please see Figure 9.5 to view all four lines. The spinolaminar (posterior margin of the spinal canal) line may have a slight step at C2 posteriorly in children but should not exceed 2 mm. All the lines should follow the normal cervical lordotic curve with no breaks in the lines or stair stepping (step-off), which may be indicative of a ligamentous injury or occult fracture. There may be straightening of the cervical lordotic curve that can be normal or from muscle spasm.

Next, the *b*one structures need to be evaluated in detail. Each vertebra from C2 downward should be rectangular in shape and similar in size

FIGURE 9.5 Four anatomical lines.
Note: A = anterior vertebral, B = posterior vertebral, C = spinolaminar, and D = posterior spinous process.
Courtesy of Theresa M. Campo.

with the anterior aspect being of similar height to the posterior aspect. If the anterior aspect is greater than 3 mm narrower than the posterior aspect, then a wedge fracture should be suspected. The normal bone structures of the cervical spine are outlined in Figure 9.6. Note the pedicles, facet joint, lamina, spinous process, and lateral mass.

(A)

(B)

FIGURE 9.6 Cervical vertebra C1 through the top of T1 (A). Note the shape and alignment of each vertebra. Normal cervical bone structures (B). Note the lateral mass, facet joint, lamina, and spinous process in addition to the vertebral bodies.
Courtesy of Theresa M. Campo.

The cartilaginous spaces are evaluated next. The area between the dens, a projection of the axis of C2, and the body of C1 is known as the predental space and should not measure more than 3 mm in an adult or 5 mm in children (Figure 9.7). If the predental space is greater than specified, then a fracture to the odontoid process or disruption of the transverse ligament

FIGURE 9.7 Predental space.
Courtesy of Theresa M. Campo.

should be suspected. If either is suspected, further imaging with either CT or MRI should be performed.

The disc space should be similar anteriorly and posteriorly between each vertebrae and similar in height along the cervical spine. Decreases in disc space may occur from degenerative changes. However, if a decrease in height is noted, an MRI should be considered to evaluate the possibility of a disc herniation.

The nasopharyngeal, retropharyngeal, and retrotracheal space should be evaluated for Soft tissue swelling (Figure 9.8). The nasopharyngeal space anterior to C1 should not measure more than 10 mm. The retropharyngeal space anterior to C2 to C3/C4 should measure between 4 and 7 mm and the retrotracheal space anterior to C5 to C7 should not exceed 14 mm in children and 22 mm in adults. Increased measurements in these areas may be indicative of a vertebral fracture causing bleeding or hematoma formation and requires further imaging.

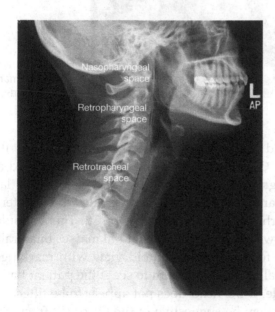

FIGURE 9.8 Nasopharyngeal, retropharyngeal, and retrotracheal spaces.
Courtesy of Theresa M. Campo.

The AP view is often overlooked but valuable in identifying some fractures better than are seen on the lateral view. After determining adequacy, alignment should be evaluated by looking at vertebral body edges and the articular pillars. The spinal processes should be midline and aligned in the vertical plane. If malalignment is identified, and the patient's head is not turned or shifted, a facet joint dislocation should be suspected. Each cervical vertebral body height and the intervertebral joint spaces should also be equal. The distance between the spinous processes in the vertical plane should also be equal. If the space between the spinous processes exceeds more than half the width of the vertebral body above or below, suspect an anterior cervical dislocation. Please see Figure 9.9 for a normal AP view with markings.

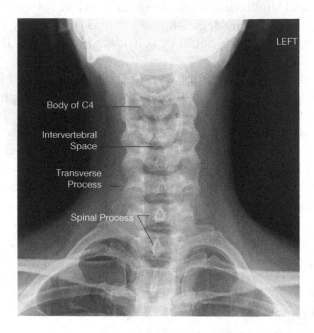

FIGURE 9.9 Anterior–posterior view with markings.
Courtesy of Theresa M. Campo.

The odontoid view is considered to be adequate if it allows for visualization of C1 and C2, including the entire odontoid and lateral borders of C1. Alignment of the occipital condyle with the lateral mass and superior articular facet of C1 should be visualized. The lateral masses of C1 should not overhang the lateral masses of C2. There should be symmetry of the space between the dens in the lateral masses bilaterally of C1. Please see Figure 9.10 for a normal odontoid view with markings. If the spaces are asymmetrical, evaluate the film to see if the patient has his or her head tilted to one side. If the head does not appear to be tilted to one side, then the asymmetry may be suggestive of the C1 or C2 fracture. The odontoid should blend with the body of C2 and should not have any disruptions of the cortical margins. If there is disruption of the cortical margins, then a fracture should be suspected.

Soft tissue, tooth shadows, or the occiput can produce shadows that may mimic a fracture. To avoid this mistake, outline the shadow that is going through the odontoid to see if it progresses past the cortical margins of the odontoid itself. If you are able to discern an absolute outline of an underlying or overlapping structure, no further imaging is necessary. However, if you are not able to do this or there is any question whatsoever, further imaging should be done.

(A)

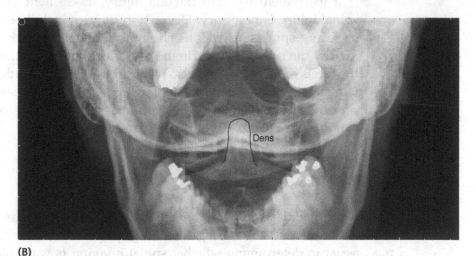

(B)

FIGURE 9.10 Odontoid view with markings (A); dens (B).
Courtesy of Theresa M. Campo.

If pain persists and no abnormalities are identified on the routine three views, additional views such as oblique as well as flexion and extension can be considered. Oblique views are taken at a 45° angle and can increase visibility of the intervertebral foramina in the presence of spondylosis of the facet joints. The right posterior oblique demonstrates the left foramina and the right anterior oblique demonstrates the right foramina.

Flexion and extension views are used to visualize ligament instability and to assess vertebral mobility. If mild malalignment is identified on routine views, the flexion and extension is especially useful in the trauma patient to rule out ligamentous injury when there is minimal malalignment seen on plain radiographs.

Cervical spine trauma is most often seen with the cervical spine in hyperflexion. This is because when the head is flexed the force exerts itself on the C4 through C7 vertebral bodies, causing compression of the vertebral bodies and anterior wedging. In the posterior aspect, the lamina within the spinal processes and the supporting ligaments may be placed in tension, resulting in fracture and tears. Hyperextension injuries are less common, occurring only 20% of the time. These injuries result from tension on the anterior longitudinal ligament which may tear at the margin of the vertebral body or the intervertebral disc space. Hyperextension injuries may include avulsion fractures when the vertebral body is affected, fracture of the spinal processes posteriorly, and fracture of the lamina and facets. Axial trauma can cause compression to the intervertebral disc causing comminuted vertebral body fractures.

If the patient has a distraction injury, assessment for head trauma or spinal injury is necessary. Distraction injuries include extremity fractures or severe sprains, as well as chest, abdominal, or back trauma. Rotation injuries can cause fractures in the posterior elements of the spine, especially the facets and lamina, and also result in fracture dislocation. Always maintain stability of the cervical spine if injury is strongly suspected by using cervical immobilization devices such as a cervical collar, cervical immobilization device (CID), or equivalent equipment.

ABNORMALITIES

Abnormalities can occur anywhere along the cervical spine and involve either bone fracture or ligamentous injury. Using the NEXUS or CCR can assist in determining whether spinal imaging is warranted in identifying abnormalities. Any injury to the upper cervical area can be life-threatening and must be identified as soon as possible. Most cervical fractures occur between C3 and C7.

A Jefferson fracture occurs from compression of the bony ring of the C1 vertebra (Figure 9.11). This is usually caused by an axial load to the vertex of the head, usually from a diving injury. The fracture involves the anterior and posterior arches of C1 bilaterally with displacement of the C1 lateral masses beyond the margin of the body of C2. If lateral displacement is more than 2 mm or if unilateral displacement occurs, a C1 fracture may be present. If this is suspected, a CT scan is required to identify and delineate the extent of the fracture and possible impingement. Jefferson fractures are considered to be unstable and must be addressed immediately to avoid devastating neurological and life-threatening sequelae.

(A)

(B)

(C)

FIGURE 9.11 Jefferson fracture on radiograph (A); drawing depicting the injury (B); the fracture on CT scan slice (C).

(*continued*)

(D)

FIGURE 9.11 (*continued*) Drawing depicting the injury (D).
Source: University of Virginia. Permission granted by the University of Virginia Department of Radiology and Medical Imaging.

Fractures to the odontoid are best seen on the lateral view and are suspected with an anterior tilt or movement of the odontoid. This may be the only sign of a fracture and may be accompanied by prevertebral soft tissue swelling. Odontoid fractures are divided into three types. Type I is a fracture of the superior tip of the odontoid. It is relatively rare and can potentially be unstable. Type II odontoid fractures occur at the base of the odontoid, are the most common type, and are considered to be unstable. Type III odontoid fractures occur through the base of the odontoid into the body of the axis and have the best prognosis. Please see Figure 9.12 for the three types of odontoid fractures.

(A1)

FIGURE 9.12 Type I odontoid fracture (A1).

(*continued*)

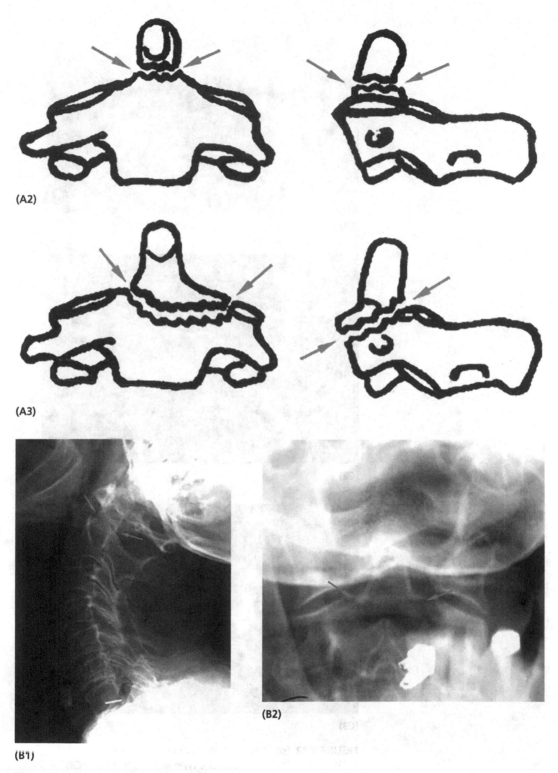

(A2)

(A3)

(B1)

(B2)

FIGURE 9.12 (*continued*) Type II odontoid fracture (A2); type III odontoid fracture (A3); type II dens fracture lateral view (B1); type II dens fracture odontoid view (B2).

(*continued*)

(C1)

(C2)

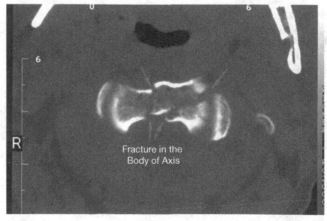

(C3)

FIGURE 9.12 (*continued*) Type III dens fracture odontoid view (C1); type III dens fracture (C2); type III dens fracture (C3). Note clarity with CT image.
Source: University of Virginia. Permission granted by the University of Virginia Department of Radiology and Medical Imaging.

A fracture through the pars interarticularis of the axis of C2 is known as a hangman's fracture (Figure 9.13). This fracture occurs from hyperextension such as in a motor vehicle accident when the head hits the dashboard. This fracture is accompanied by prevertebral soft tissue swelling and avulsion of the anterior inferior corner of C2. Additionally, there may be rupture of the anterior longitudinal ligament, anterior dislocation of the C2 vertebral body, and bilateral pars interarticularis fractures. A hangman's fracture is considered to be unstable and is best seen on the lateral view.

FIGURE 9.13 • Hangman's fracture.
Courtesy of Dr. Douglas W. Parrillo.

A teardrop fracture occurs when there is an anterior compression fracture of the vertebral body resulting from a severe flexion injury, such as diving into shallow water (Figure 9.14). There may also be posterior ligament disruption as well as prevertebral swelling associated with the anterior longitudinal ligament tear. This avulsion fracture from the anterior vertebral body resembles a teardrop on the lateral view. There may also be posterior vertebral body subluxation into the spinal canal with spinal cord compression and instability. This injury may also be accompanied by a fracture of the spinous process as well as vertebral body displacement and is considered to be unstable.

FIGURE 9.14 Teardrop fracture.
Courtesy of Dr. Douglas W. Parrillo.

Complete anterior dislocation of the vertebral body resulting from extreme flexion of the head and neck without axial compression results in bilateral facet dislocation, is considered unstable, and is associated with a high risk for spinal cord damage. There may be complete anterior dislocation of the vertebral body by half its AP diameter. Disruption of the posterior and anterior longitudinal ligament may accompany this injury, causing a bowtie or batwing appearance of the locked facets. This injury is best seen on the lateral view (see Figure 9.15).

X-TABLE
4:20 PM
WJ

FIGURE 9.15 Bilateral facet dislocation.
Courtesy of Dr. Douglas W. Parrillo.

In contrast, a unilateral facet dislocation and rupture of the apophyseal joint ligaments can be seen with an anterior dislocation of the affected vertebral body by less than half of the vertebral body AP diameter. There may also be discordant rotation above and below the involved level as well as the facet within the intervertebral foramina, which is best seen as a widening of the disc space on the oblique. Again, a bowtie or batwing appearance of the overriding locked facet may occur. This injury is considered to be stable and occurs from flexion and rotation simultaneously occurring. Please see Figure 9.16 showing a unilateral facet dislocation.

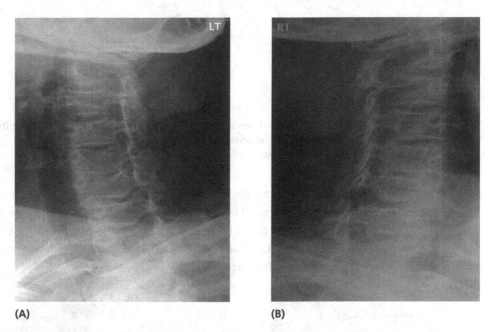

(A) **(B)**

FIGURE 9.16 (A) and (B) demonstrate unilateral locked facet with fracture.
Courtesy of Dr. Douglas W. Parrillo.

Anterior subluxation occurs when there is disruption of the posterior ligamentous complex with loss of normal cervical lordosis and anterior displacement of the vertebral body accompanied by fanning of the interspinous distance. This is considered to be unstable if the anterior subluxation is more than 4 mm with an associated compression fracture of more than 20% of the affected vertebral body height, an increase or decrease in normal disc space, and if fanning occurs of the interspinous distance. This may be difficult to diagnose because of muscle spasms presenting similarly. This injury may be considered to be stable initially but then becomes unstable 20% to 50% of the time with hyperflexion of the neck. Please see Figure 9.17 for anterior subluxation.

Clay shoveler's fracture is a fracture of the C6 to T1 spinal process. This injury is often caused by hyperflexion with contraction of the paraspinous

FIGURE 9.17 Normal cervical spine (A); anterior subluxation C spine (B). Note the mal alignment of the anterior line.
Courtesy of Theresa M. Campo.

muscles, which avulse the spinal process itself. This fracture is best viewed in the lateral view. It is considered to be stable and may be accompanied by a ghost sign on the AP view, caused by the overlapping of the spinal processes of C6 or C7 due to the displaced fracture. Please see Figure 9.18 for clay shoveler's fracture.

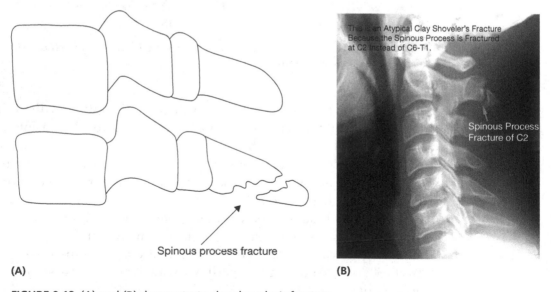

Spinous process fracture

(A)

This is an Atypical Clay Shoveler's Fracture Because the Spinous Process is Fractured at C2 Instead of C6-T1.

Spinous Process Fracture of C2

(B)

FIGURE 9.18 (A) and (B) demonstrate clay shoveler's fracture.
Source: University of Virginia. Permission granted by the University of Virginia Department of Radiology and Medical Imaging.

A compression fracture caused by hyperflexion and compression that causes buckling of the anterior cortex and loss of height of the anterior vertebral body with anterior superior fracture of the vertebral body is known as a wedge fracture (Figure 9.19). Burst fractures can occur at the levels of C3 through C7 from axial compression (Figure 9.20). This injury can cause damage to the spinal cord from the displacement of the posterior fragments and requires CT for further evaluation, although it is considered to be a stable fracture.

(A)   (B)

FIGURE 9.19 Normal cervical vertebra (A); anterior wedge compression fracture (B).
Courtesy of Theresa M. Campo.

FIGURE 9.20 Burst fracture.
Courtesy of Dr. Douglas W. Parrillo.

Atlanto-occipital dislocation is the separation of the skull from the cervical spine. This injury commonly occurs when a person is ejected from a motor vehicle, especially younger children younger than the age of 2 years (see Figure 9.21).

(A)   **(B)**

FIGURE 9.21 (A) and (B) demonstrate atlanto-occipital dislocation. Note the anterior displacement of the occipital condyles.
Source: University of Virginia. Permission granted by the University of Virginia Department of Radiology and Medical Imaging.

Osteoarthritic degenerative changes in the cervical spine occur with aging. These changes can include loss of disc height, bone spurring, and increased prevertebral space swelling, which may be normal in the aging client. These changes make it challenging to evaluate acute injuries with plain radiograph images. Therefore, imaging for acute injury using CT or MRI may be necessary to evaluate the cervical bones and to assess the spinal cord for any abnormalities, including partial compression stenosis or complete nerve root impingement.

CONCLUSION

It is important to obtain adequate films to ensure accurate interpretation of cervical spine conditions. Cervical spine radiographs may be beneficial in identifying fractures, subluxations, dislocations, and degenerative changes. Closely adhering to evidence-based guidelines such as the NEXUS and CCR criteria will reduce the likelihood of inappropriate imaging. However, the provider should remember that degenerative changes and abnormalities noted with plain films may warrant imaging with CT or MRI to avoid missing potentially life-threatening or debilitating spinal cord trauma.

RESOURCES

Au-Yong, I., Au-Yong, A., & Broderick, N. (2010). *On-call x-rays made easy*. Philadelphia, PA: Churchill Livingstone, Elsevier.

Barakos, J. A., & Purcell, D. D. (2012). Head and neck imaging. In W. E. Brant & C. A. Helms (Eds.), *Fundamentals of diagnostic radiology* (4th ed., pp. 240–266). Philadelphia, PA: Wolters Kluwer/Lippincott Williams & Wilkins.

Daffner, R. H. (2014). Musculoskeletal imaging. In R. H. Daffner & M. S. Hartman (Eds.), *Clinical radiology: The essentials* (4th ed., pp. 482–533). Philadelphia, PA: Wolters Kluwer/Lippincott Williams & Wilkins.

Herring, W. (2016). *Learning radiology: Recognizing the basics* (3rd ed., pp. 266–278). Philadelphia, PA: Elsevier.

Yao, L. L., Gay, S. B., Vu, Q. D. M., Anderson, M. W., Powell, S. M., & Patel, P. N. (n.d.). Imaging evaluation of the cervical spine. Retrieved from https://www.med-ed.virginia.edu/courses/rad/cspine/index.html

Basic Interpretation of Thoracic Spine Radiographs

Numerous conditions can predispose a person to a spinal injury, including degeneration, malignancy, loss of bone density, Paget's disease, autoimmune disorders, hemorrhagic disease, and congenital disorders or malformations. The thoracic spine is generally better protected than the cervical spine and greater forces are needed to cause serious injury. Because of this, injuries of the thoracic spine may be associated with additional injuries of the chest and abdomen, including rib fractures and abdominal organ injuries. Remember to always protect the spine during assessment by maintaining alignment and stabilization and to treat life-threatening injuries first.

Thoracic spine injuries should be suspected in patients who present after a fall, have multiple injuries, have a neurological deficit, or have a mechanism of severe local force. Injuries should also be suspected in patients with fractures to the sternum, the ribs, or the scapula. In patients who are elderly or have osteoporosis, it may not take a great deal of force to cause a wedge or compression fracture in the thoracic spine. In fact, simply rolling over in bed may cause a compression fracture with severe osteoporosis. In general, most fractures of the thoracic spine occur in the lower two thirds.

NORMAL

Thoracic radiographs generally involve two views: the anterior–posterior (AP) view and the lateral view. Adequate films require that the lower cervical (top of C7) and upper lumbar spine (top of L2) are included on both views (Figure 10.1). When evaluating the AP and lateral views, there should be symmetry in the height of each of the vertebrae and equal spacing between the vertebrae and spinal processes. However, it is important to note that the vertebral body and intervertebral disc spaces become slightly larger at the base of the thoracic spine at the junction with the lumbar spine (T12 and L1).

(A)

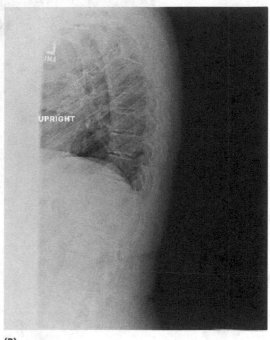

(B)

FIGURE 10.1 Anterior–posterior view T spine (A); lateral view T spine (B).
Source: Radiograph.

When evaluating the AP view, the pedicle, spinous process, and transverse process should be easily visualized (Figure 10.2). On the lateral view, one should visualize the vertebral bodies and pedicles (Figure 10.3). When reviewing thoracic spine images, view the outline of each vertebral body, pedicle, and transverse and spinal process systematically. Evaluate the distance between the pedicles as well as the vertebral disc spaces. The vertebral bodies should have smooth margins from the base of the cervical spine through the top of the lumbar spine. Any disruptions in alignment and/or disc spaces may be indicative of injury.

Adequacy of the images should be ensured prior to interpretation as with any other radiograph. Evaluating alignment begins with the spinal processes. They should be readily visible on the AP view from the base

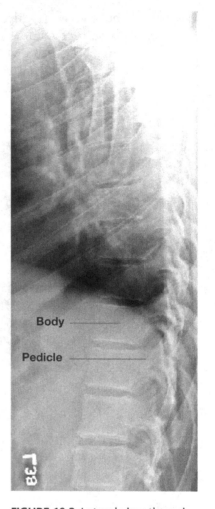

FIGURE 10.2 Anterior–posterior view thoracic spine with markings.
Source: University of Virginia.
Permission granted by the University of Virginia Department of Radiology and Medical Imaging.

FIGURE 10.3 Lateral view thoracic spine with markings.
Source: University of Virginia.
Permission granted by the University of Virginia Department of Radiology and Medical Imaging.

of the cervical spine through to T4 or T5 and then again at the lower end of the thoracic spine. Both the anterior and posterior margins of the vertebra should be in alignment on the lateral view. The vertebral *b*one (body) should have uniform margins that are aligned with no interruption in the margins. The pedicles should also be visualized on the lateral view without any disruptions along their borders. It is important to note that in the lateral view the first four vertebral bodies are not readily visible because they are obscured by the shoulder girdle and superimposed ribs, as well as lung markings. There is no "*C*" when interpreting the thoracic spine. The intervertebral *d*isc spaces should get progressively larger with progression toward the lumbar spine. The paravertebral *S*oft tissue line may be visible and is considered normal. However, any enhancement and/or displacement of this line may be indicative of swelling and an injury. See Figures 10.4 and 10.5 for interpretation of the thoracic spine.

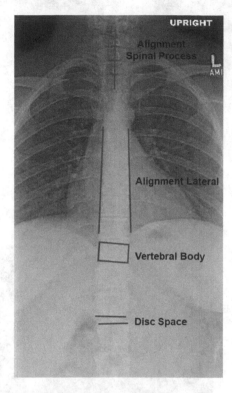

FIGURE 10.4 Anterior–posterior view interpretation.
Courtesy of Dr. David Begleiter; diagramming, Theresa M. Campo.

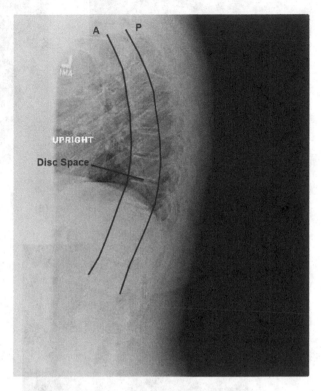

FIGURE 10.5 Lateral view interpretation.
Courtesy of Dr. David Begleiter; diagramming, Theresa M. Campo.

ABNORMALITIES

There are three common mechanisms that cause injury to the thoracic spine: hyperflexion, vertical compression, and shearing injury. The most common of these is hyperflexion, which causes anterior compression of the vertebral body known as wedging. See Figure 10.6 demonstrating anterior compression or wedge fracture.

Vertical compression can cause loss of height to the vertebral body in a crushing manner. See Figure 10.7, which demonstrates a compression fracture. The severity of the compression to the vertebra may vary. There is a natural tapering of the anterior thoracic vertebral body that should not be confused with a compression fracture where there is loss of height as well as disruption of the posterior line. Compression fractures are more common in women than men and may occur secondary to osteoporosis with minimal force.

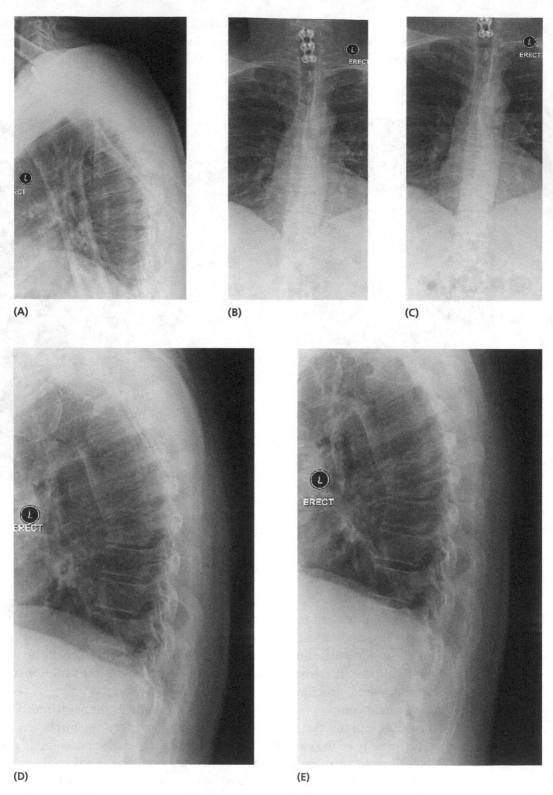

FIGURE 10.6 (A) through (E) demonstrate anterior wedge fracture.
Courtesy of Dr. David Parrillo.

(A)   (B)

FIGURE 10.7 (A) and (B) demonstrate thoracic compression fracture. Note compressed look to vertebra compared with surrounding vertebrae.
Source: University of Virginia. Permission granted by the University of Virginia Department of Radiology and Medical Imaging.

A high-energy axial load can cause the disc above a vertebra to be driven downward, causing the vertebra to burst. This may cause fragments to be pushed into the spinal canal (retropulsed). This is known as a burst fracture (Figure 10.8) and may involve one or more vertebra. Burst fractures are commonly associated with neurological deficits due to the fragments being retropulsed into the spinal canal. This injury usually occurs from a motor vehicle crash or a fall.

(A)   (B)

FIGURE 10.8 Burst fracture (A); burst fracture CT scan three-dimentional reconstruction (B).
Courtesy of Dr. Douglas W. Parrillo.

A chance fracture can occur from wearing a lap belt or when children are not properly restrained in a correct child safety seat during a motor vehicle crash. Chance fractures are transverse fractures through the vertebral body, pedicle, and spinal process. This fracture is most commonly seen in the lower thoracic and upper lumbar spine and may be associated with intra-abdominal injury (Figure 10.9).

FIGURE 10.9 Chance fracture. Reprinted by permission of James Heilman, MD, Wikipedian, ER Department Head, East Kootenay Regional Hospital, Clinical Assistant Professor, Department of Emergency Medicine, University of British Columbia.

CONCLUSION

When evaluating the thoracic spine, it is important to make sure that there is proper alignment, bone integrity, and disc space. This can be evaluated on both the AP and lateral views. Although the thoracic spine is better protected than the cervical spine, it still has the potential for significant fracture and injury that may result in loss of function.

RESOURCES

Au-Yong, I., Au-Yong, A., & Broderick, N. (2010). *On-call x-rays made easy*. Philadelphia, PA: Churchill Livingstone, Elsevier.

Daffner, R. H. (2014). Musculoskeletal imaging. In D. H. Daffner & M. S. Hartman (Eds.), *Clinical radiology: The essentials* (4th ed., pp. 482–533). Philadelphia, PA: Wolters Kluwer/Lippincott Williams & Wilkins.

Helms, C. A. (2012). Lumbar spine: Disc disease and stenosis. In W. E. Brant & C. A. Helms (Eds.), *Fundamentals of diagnostic radiology* (4th ed., pp. 314–323). Philadelphia, PA: Wolters Kluwer/Lippincott Williams & Wilkins.

Herring, W. (2016). *Learning radiology: Recovering the basics* (3rd ed., pp. 266–278). Philadelphia, PA: Elsevier.

Kuntz, A. F., Lai, W. S., Norton, P. T., Yao, L. L., & Gay, S. B. (n.d.). Skeletal trauma. Retrieved from https://www.med-ed.virginia.edu/courses/rad/ext/index.html

11

Basic Interpretation of Lumbar Spine Radiographs

There are many similarities between the thoracic and lumbar spine. They are both better protected than the cervical spine; as a result, it can take a great deal of force to cause injury. As with thoracic spine injuries, lumbar spine injuries are often associated with injuries to the abdomen and pelvis and pelvic structures. Acute back pain can result from either fracture, sprain, or strain. It may also be caused by degenerative changes, overuse injuries, infection, or a herniated nucleus pulposus (HNP) or herniated disc.

NORMAL

When evaluating the lumbar spine, there are two main views that are obtained; the anterior–posterior (AP) and the lateral views (Figure 11.1). Lumbar spine images should include the upper level of T10 if traumatic injury is suspected. Most lumbar injuries, approximately two thirds, occur at the level of T12 to L2, which is why imaging T10 and T11 is necessary.

While evaluating the AP and lateral views of the lumbar spine, carefully inspect the vertebral bodies, spinous and transverse processes, and pedicles

FIGURE 11.1 (A) through (C) demonstrate normal lumbar spine views.
Source: Radiograph.

on the AP view. On the lateral view, examine the inferior articular and superior articular processes. These areas are shown in Figure 11.2.

The vertebral bodies of the lumbar region have a slight increase in height as you move downward toward the sacrum. The vertebral bodies should have smooth margins and be in full alignment. The disc spaces also have a slight increase as you move down, but the disc space of L5–S1 is slightly

FIGURE 11.2 (A) through (E) demonstrate normal views with markings.
Source: Radiograph.

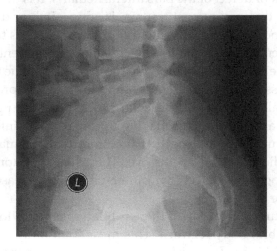

FIGURE 11.3 (A) through (C) demonstrate the L-spine with disc spaces. A, anterior; L, lateral; P, posterior; SP, spinal process.
Source: Radiopaediageneral@radiopaedia.org

less than the disc space of L4–L5. As with any other radiograph, you want to make sure that you are evaluating the entire image from left to right and from top to bottom.

Adequacy of the images should be evaluated and be acceptable. Alignment on the AP view should be evaluated using the spinal processes to ensure that they line up as well as the lateral borders of the vertebral bodies and pedicles. On the lateral view, alignment is assessed by viewing the anterior and posterior margins of the vertebral bodies and ensuring that they line up to one another. Each vertebral body from T11 through to the sacrum should be evaluated on both views for cortical disruptions indicative of fracture. Evaluation of the intervertebral disc spaces should be evaluated next, which should be approximately equal with the exception of L5–S1; this is slightly less than L4–L5. Evaluate the space between the pedicles as well as the soft tissue lines for any increased space that may indicate swelling or hematoma formation from the injury. The majority of abnormalities of the lumbar spine can be identified on the lateral view. Please view Figure 11.3 for the ABCDs (adequacy and alignment, body, cartilage or joints, disc space, soft tissue) of the L-spine.

ABNORMALITIES

The majority of injuries to the lumbar spine are quite similar to those found in the thoracic spine. The majority of injuries to the lumbar spine occur between the area of T12 and L2 and include compression, wedge, and chance fractures. Degenerative changes can also cause back pain and can be identified on plain radiographs, as can spondylolysis, spondylolisthesis, and spinal stenosis.

Spondylolysis is a break or defect of the pars interarticularis. It is thought to be a chronic condition that occurs post trauma, is congenital, or develops after a fall to the buttocks during early childhood, causing stress to the lumbar spine. It most often occurs at the level of L5 and can be identified on radiograph as a "Scottie dog" figure. This is best seen on an oblique view with the transverse process making up the nose, superior articular process making up the ear, contralateral superior articular process making up the tail, contralateral inferior articular process making up the rear leg, inferior articular process making up the front leg, the pars interarticularis making up the neck, and the pedicle making up the eye. The collar that appears around the neck of the dog is the defect that can be visualized. Please see Figure 11.4 for the "Scottie dog" figure.

Spondylolisthesis (Figure 11.5) occurs if there is bilateral spondylolysis with shifting of the vertebral body forward. This most commonly occurs at the level of L4–L5 and L5–S1. If severe, there can be neural foraminal

Nose: *transverse process*

Ear: *superior articular process*

Eye: *pedicle*

Tail: *contralateral superior articular process*

Neck: *pars interarticularis*

Body: *lamina*

Front leg: *inferior articular process*

Rear leg: *contralateral inferior articular process*

(A1)

(A2)

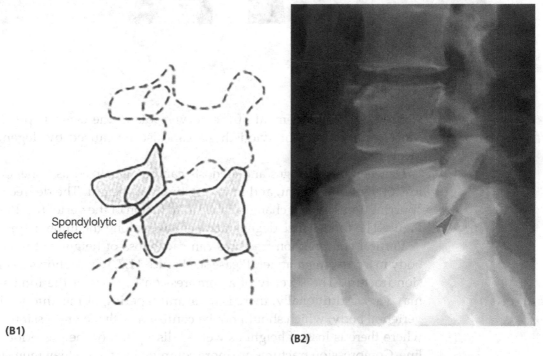

Spondylolytic defect

(B1)

(B2)

FIGURE 11.4 Scottie dog model of lumbar spine (A1 and A2); Spondylolysis (B1 and B2).
Source: University of Virginia. Permission granted by the University of Virginia Department of Radiology and Medical Imaging.

FIGURE 11.5 Spondylolisthesis.
Courtesy of Dr. Douglas W. Parrillo.

stenosis and impingement of the nerve roots in the central spinal canal. More commonly, spondylolisthesis can also be caused by degenerative facet changes.

Degenerative changes and stenosis can be visualized as bone spurring, loss of vertebral height, and intravertebral disc height. The degree of bone spurring and sclerotic changes can lead to fusion of the vertebrae. Please see Figure 11.6 to visualize degenerative changes along the lumbar spine.

Vertical compression fractures can cause loss of height to the vertebral body in a crushing manner. Please see Figure 11.7, which shows a compression fracture. The severity of a compression fracture of the lumbar spine may vary. Additionally, there is a natural tapering of the anterior lumbar vertebral body, which should not be confused with a compression fracture where there is loss of height as well as disruption of the posterior cortical line. Compression fractures are more common in women than men and may occur secondary to osteoporosis with minimal force. They most frequently occur in the upper lumbar region and at the thoraco-lumbar junction

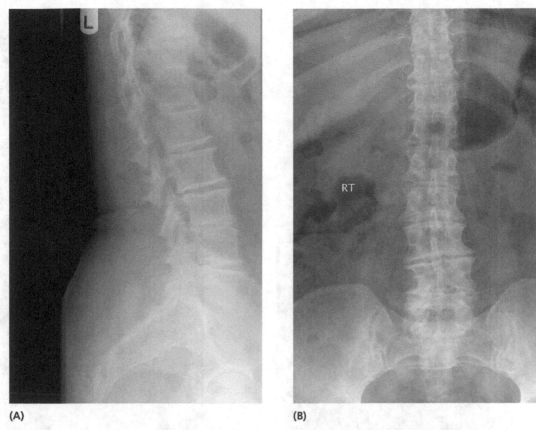

(A) (B)

FIGURE 11.6 Degeneration of the lumbar spine (A). Note lack of clarity vertebral bodies and development of osteophytes. Degeneration of the lumbar spine (B). Note loss of vertebral body shape. Courtesy of Dr. Douglas W. Parrillo.

specifically. Anterior wedge fractures may also be identified but are more common at the thoraco-lumbar junction. Further evaluation may be required with CT scan or MRI to identify associated spinal canal injuries or if there is a strong suspicion of a fracture based on the history and physical; these signs may not show up on the plain radiograph.

Lumbar chance fractures, like thoracic chance fractures, can occur from wearing a lap belt during a motor vehicle crash or may occur in children who are not restrained in a weight-appropriate child restraint device. Chance fractures that are transverse fractures through the vertebral body, pedicle, and spinal process are most commonly seen in the lower thoracic and upper lumbar spine and may be associated with intra-abdominal injury (Figure 11.8).

(A)
(B)

FIGURE 11.7 Lumbar compression fracture on the anterior–posterior (A) and lateral view (B). Note the loss of vertebral height on both views and the malalignment of L4, L5, S1 on the lateral view. There is also a bone fragment visualized in the lateral view.
Source: University of Virginia. Permission granted by the University of Virginia Department of Radiology and Medical Imaging.

Traumatic injuries can cause fractures to the vertebral body and the pedicle as well as the spinous and transverse processes. It is important to evaluate all bony margins at all levels of the lower thoracic, lumbar, and sacrum. Evaluation of the lower ribs as well as the sacrum is imperative to ensure no fractures to any bony structures. See Figure 11.9 for various L-spine fractures.

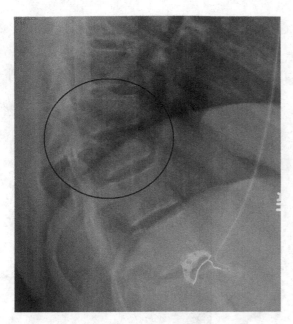

FIGURE 11.8 Chance fracture.
Reprinted by permission of James Heilman, MD, Wikipedian, ER Department Head, East Kootenay Regional Hospital, Clinical Assistant Professor, Department of Emergency Medicine, University of British Columbia.

(A)

(B)

FIGURE 11.9 (A) through (D) demonstrate coccyx fracture.

(continued)

(C)   (D)

FIGURE 11.9 (*continued*)
Courtesy of Dr. Douglas W. Parrillo.

CONCLUSION

Fractures and chronic changes of the lumbar spine can be easily identified on plain radiographs. However, if a fracture is suspected and not visualized on a plain radiograph, further study may be required for evaluation of occult fractures and soft tissue injuries. Overlying bowel contents and gas can further obscure structures of the lumbar spine or suggest a fracture line. When present, either repeat the image or follow up with a CT scan to rule out a fracture.

RESOURCES

Au-Yong, I., Au-Yong, A., & Broderick, N. (2010). *On-call x-rays made easy.* Philadelphia, PA: Churchill Livingstone, Elsevier.

Daffner, R. H. (2014). Musculoskeletal imaging. In D. H. Daffner & M. S. Hartman (Eds.), *Clinical radiology: The essentials* (4th ed., pp. 482–533). Philadelphia, PA: Wolters Kluwer/Lippincott Williams & Wilkins.

Helms, C. A. (2012). Lumbar spine: Disc disease and stenosis. In W. E. Brant & C. A. Helms (Eds.), *Fundamentals of diagnostic radiology* (4th ed., pp. 314–323). Philadelphia, PA: Wolters Kluwer/Lippincott Williams & Wilkins.

Herring, W. (2016). *Learning radiology: Recognizing the basics* (3rd ed., pp. 266–278). Philadelphia, PA: Elsevier.

Kuntz, A. F., Lai, W. S., Norton, P. T., Yao, L. L., & Gay, S. B. (n.d.). *Skeletal trauma*. Retrieved from https://www.med-ed.virginia.edu/courses/rad/ext/index.html

Index

Printed in the United States
By Bookmasters